CACMA Exam Practice Questions

Copyright © 2025 Examelot

All rights reserved.

No part of this book may be reproduced, stored in a retrieval system, or transmitted in any form or by any means, electronic, mechanical, photocopying, recording, or otherwise, without the prior written permission of the author.

First published in 2024

This edition was published on September 17, 2025

This work is not created or endorsed by the California Certifying Board for Medical Assistants (CCBMA)

Visit Examelot's site at **examelot.com**

ISBN 9798327105522

CACMA Exam Practice Questions

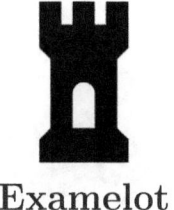

Examelot

Preface

Contents

About the CACMA exam 3

Practice questions 9
    Content Area 1: Scrubbing Patient Charts 10
        Answers *13*
    Content Area 2: Checking-In Patients 15
        Answers *19*
    Content Area 3: Rooming Patients 21
        Answers *27*
    Content Area 4: Collecting Patient Vitals 30
        Answers *38*
    Content Area 5: Performing Point of Care Orders 42
        Answers *63*
    Content Area 6: Administering Medications/Vaccines 74
        Answers *84*
    Content Area 7: Discharging Patients 90
        Answers *94*
    Content Area 8: Responding to Codes/Emergencies 96
        Answers *102*
    Content Area 9: Managing Communication 107
        Answers *111*

Hi! I'm Merlin, the Question Master of Examelot. Welcome to this study guide and question book for the CACMA exam!

This book contains 300 practice questions for the CACMA exam, divided into the nine content areas of the exam. You can find the answers at the end of each section.

If you have any issues or concerns, send the Examelot team an email at **contact@examelot.com**.

Good luck in your CACMA exam!

Merlin

About the CACMA exam

Introduction

The California Certified Medical Assistant (CACMA) examination assesses the skills and knowledge required of entry-level medical assistants. The exam is set by the California Certifying Board for Medical Assistants (CCBMA).

Passing the CACMA exam earns you a certificate and allows you to use the CACMA credential after your name.

Exam eligibility

Before applying for the CACMA exam, ensure you meet the eligibility criteria.

The exam has six eligibility routes:

1. Currently employed as a medical assistant in the U.S.
2. Graduated from a medical assisting program in the U.S. within the last five years
3. Worked full-time as a medical assistant in the U.S. for at least two years within the last five years
4. Working as a medical assisting instructor in an accredited institution in the U.S.
5. Served in the U.S. military as a medical assistant in the last year
6. Served in the U.S. military as a medical assistant for at least two of the past five years

Additionally, you must have training in venipuncture and/or administering injections (documented by a signed Certificate of Competency) and hold current CPR certification.

Applying for the CACMA exam

You can apply for the CACMA exam online at ccbma.org by following these steps:

1. Go to ccbma.org
2. Click *Get Certified*
3. Under *Apply for the Exam*, select *Begin*
4. Fill in your personal details
5. Create a CCBMA account using the link the CCBMA emails to you
6. Upload the required documents and pay the $250 exam fee

The CCBMA will process your application within 15 business days. Once approved, you can schedule your exam at a Pearson VUE testing center.

Documents you'll need to apply

You'll need the following documents to apply for the CACMA exam:

- Photo ID (driver's license, state ID card, or passport)
- CPR card or Basic Life Support (BLS) card
- Statement of Proficiency form (if you're applying as an employee or graduate). The form must completed and signed by a doctor, nurse, or physician assistant
- Proof of employment (if you're applying as an employee)
- Certificate of Completion (if you're applying as a graduate)
- Discharge form DD214 (if you're applying as an ex-member of the US military)

Rescheduling the exam

Contact Pearson VUE if you need to reschedule your exam. Rescheduling is free if you do it more than 24 hours in advance. However, if you reschedule within 24 hours of the exam start time, you will be charged a same-day forfeit exam fee.

Cancelling the exam

If you need to cancel a scheduled exam, contact Pearson VUE and CCBMA at least 15 days before the exam. CCBMA will refund your testing fee minus a $75 processing charge.

If you haven't scheduled your exam yet, you can cancel directly with CCBMA. They will cancel your application and refund your testing fee minus a $75 processing charge.

What to bring to the exam

You must bring a government ID with your photo and signature, such as a driver's license, a state identity card, a passport, or a military ID.

You are *not* allowed to bring into the exam room:

- calculators (the test center will provide a calculator on request)
- phones
- books, notes, or paper
- food or drinks

You'll be given a locker to store these items.

Exam day

On the exam day, arrive at the testing center at least 30 minutes before the exam starts to allow time to check in and show your ID.

You'll be given a locker to store your belongings. You'll then be taken to a computer where you'll do the exam. The exam is 3 hours and 30 minutes long, with no breaks. You can change and review your answers before final submission.

How do I get my results?

After you finish the exam, the computer will tell you if you passed or failed.

If you pass, the CCBMA will mail your certificate, wallet card, and pin to you within 4 weeks.

What if I fail the exam?

If you fail the CACMA exam, don't worry! There is no limit to the number of times you can take the exam, which means you can keep retaking it until you pass. However, you will need to pay the exam fee of $250 for each retake.

Recertification

The CACMA credential expires after five years. To recertify, you must:

- pay a recertification fee of $200
- accumulate 60 continuing education units (CEUs)

The CEUs must be relevant to medical assisting and include training in CPR, HIPAA, and Cultural Competency. Visit the CCBMA website (ccbma.org) for more information on earning and counting CEUs.

Exam structure

The CACMA exam consists of 160 multiple-choice questions across nine content areas:

Content area	% of exam
A. Scrubbing patient charts	3%
B. Checking-in patients	5%
C. Rooming patients	12%
D. Collecting patient vitals	16%
E. Performing point of care orders	25%
F. Administering medications/vaccines	16%
G. Discharging patients	5%
H. Responding to codes/emergencies	13%
I. Managing communication	5%

Content Area A. Scrubbing patient charts

The first content area of the CACMA exam, *Scrubbing patient charts*, is the least important as it is only worth 3% of the exam. This content area includes questions about:

- Determining the reason for the patient's visit
- Locating the patient's medical records
- Reviewing the doctor's assessment and plan from the patient's previous visit
- Determining if any health maintenance items are due

- Confirming the patient's insurance and/or payment method
- Confirming the appointment

Content Area B. Checking-in patients

The second content area of the CACMA exam, *Checking-in patients*, is worth 5% of the exam and includes questions about:

- Registering new patients
- Verifying patient demographics (name, date of birth, address, etc.)
- Making a copy of the patient's ID
- Obtaining the patient's insurance details
- Determining if the patient's insurance is valid
- Obtaining the patient's copay

Content Area C. Rooming patients

The third content area of the CACMA exam, *Rooming patients*, is worth 12% of the exam and includes questions about:

- Preparing the room for procedures
- Preparing the patient for procedures
- Verifying the patient's identity
- Asking the patient for their chief complaint
- Asking screening questions
- Obtaining the patient's medical history
- Reconciling medications
- Verifying pharmacy information

Content Area D. Collecting patient vitals

The fourth content area of the CACMA exam, *Collecting patient vitals*, is worth 16% of the exam and includes questions about:

- Weight and height
- Temperature
- Blood pressure
- Respiration
- Heart rate
- Oxygen level

Content Area E. Performing point of care orders

The fifth content area of the CACMA exam, *Performing point of care orders*, is the most important because it is worth 25% of the exam. It will include questions about:

- A1C test
- Blood draws
- Ear lavage
- Electrocardiograms
- Flu test
- Glucose test
- Hearing test
- Hemoglobin test
- Peak flow test
- Pregnancy test
- Purified protein derivative (PPD) test
- Strep test
- Urinalysis
- Vision test

Content Area F. Administering medications/vaccines

The sixth content area of the CACMA exam, *Administering medications/vaccines*, is worth 15% of the exam. It includes questions about:

- Verifying medication/vaccine orders
- Administering vaccines
- Administering injectables

Content Area G. Discharging patients

The seventh content area of the CACMA exam, *Discharging patients*, is worth 5% of the exam. It includes questions about:

- Giving after-visit summaries
- Giving discharge instructions
- Scheduling follow-up appointments
- Transcribing physician orders

Content Area H. Responding to codes/emergencies

The eighth content area of the CACMA exam, *Responding to codes/emergencies*, is worth 13% of the exam. It includes questions about:

- Assessing emergency situations
- Reporting emergency situations
- Controlling bleeding
- CPR
- Rapid Response Protocols (RRPs)

Content Area I. Managing communication

The final content area of the CACMA exam, *Managing communication*, is worth 5% of the exam and includes questions about:

- Managing correspondence
- Processing orders
- Processing referrals
- Processing requests for prescriptions
- Obtaining authorizations
- Obtaining physician signatures

Practice questions

Content Area 1

Scrubbing Patient Charts

There are 14 questions in this content area.

1.1 What should you do when you find a document in the wrong record?
 a) Advise the patient's doctor
 b) Destroy the document and complete an incident report
 c) Leave the document in the record
 d) Refile the document in the correct record

1.2 A hospital uses a terminal digit filing system. To find record 12-08-35, which number(s) would you use first?
 a) 08
 b) 35
 c) 12
 d) 5

1.3 Where would you find information about a patient's diet, sleep patterns, and exercise patterns?
 a) Admission form
 b) History
 c) Operative note
 d) Physical exam

Answers on page 13

1.4 How often should adults get a tetanus booster shot?
   a) Every 10 years
   b) Every 15 years
   c) Every 20 years
   d) Every 25 years

1.5 A patient calls the clinic with a life-threatening emergency. Which action should the medical assistant take?
   a) Advise the patient to call 911
   b) Book the patient into the next possible appointment
   c) Give first aid instructions over the phone
   d) Tell the patient to come in right away

1.6 Which appointment slot is best for fasting patients?
   a) First thing in the morning
   b) Late morning
   c) Mid-afternoon
   d) Last appointment of the day

1.7 What is the first step in verifying patient insurance?
   a) Calling the insurance company
   b) Collecting the patient's insurance information
   c) Recording the insurance information in the EMR
   d) Scheduling the patient's appointment

1.8 What should you do if a patient's credit card is declined?
   a) Ask if they have another card
   b) Call the patient's bank
   c) Cut up the card
   d) Waive the payment

1.9 What does "NSF" on a check mean?
   a) No service fee has been charged for the transaction
   b) The account has insufficient funds
   c) The check is a forgery
   d) The check was cashed at the wrong bank

Answers on page 14

1.10 What is the three or four-digit number on the back of a credit card?
   a) Card security code
   b) Credit card number
   c) Expiry date
   d) Issue date

1.11 Which document is written, dated, and signed and instructs a bank to pay the bearer a specific amount of money?
   a) Check
   b) Passbook
   c) Warrant
   d) Wire transfer

1.12 Where in a SOAP note does the doctor propose a treatment plan?
   a) Subjective
   b) Objective
   c) Assessment
   d) Plan

1.13 At what age is it recommended to begin colorectal cancer screening in average-risk adults?
   a) 18
   b) 25–30
   c) 45–50
   d) 65–70

1.14 How often should women aged 45–54 receive a mammogram?
   a) Every 3 months
   b) Every 6 months
   c) Every 1 year
   d) Every 3 years

Answers on page 14

ANSWERS

1.1 d) Refile the document in the correct record

If you find a document in the wrong record, the most appropriate action is to refile it in the correct location. This ensures that the patient's medical information is accurate and accessible when needed.

1.2 b) 35

In the terminal digit filing system, the primary digits are the final numbers, the secondary digits are the middle numbers, and the tertiary digits are the first numbers. So for 12-08-35:

- Primary digits: 35 (the last two numbers)
- Secondary digits: 08 (the middle two numbers)
- Tertiary digits: 12 (the first two numbers)

To find patient record 12-08-35, you would first use the primary digits (35) to go to the correct shelving unit. Next, you would use the middle digits (08) to find the correct shelf. Finally, you would use the first two digits (12) to find the correct file.

1.3 b) History

A medical history includes information about chronic health conditions, current medications, allergies, childhood illnesses, family illnesses, surgeries, and immunizations. It may also include information about health habits, such as diet and exercise.

1.4 a) Every 10 years

Adults should get a tetanus booster vaccine every ten years, as the shot provides roughly ten years of protection.

1.5 a) Advise the patient to call 911

If a patient calls the clinic with a life-threatening emergency, the medical assistant should advise the patient to call 911 immediately. This ensures the patient will receive the fastest and most appropriate emergency medical response.

1.6 a) First thing in the morning

Fasting patients should be given the earliest appointment slot available. This allows them to fast overnight, perform the test or procedure first thing in the morning, and then resume eating normally for the rest of the day.

1.7 b) Collecting the patient's insurance information

The steps in verifying patient insurance are:

1. Collect the patient's insurance information from the patient
2. Contact the insurance company to verify the information the patient gave you
3. Record the information in the EMR

1.8 a) Ask if they have another card

if a patient's credit card is declined, you should ask if they have another card. This allows the patient a chance to complete the payment. You can also offer alternative methods of payment, like cash or checks.

Calling the patient's bank is not the responsibility of healthcare staff. This would be a private matter between the patient and their bank.

Cutting up the card is disrespectful to the patient's property and unnecessary.

1.9 b) The account has insufficient funds

Banks will return checks when there are insufficient funds in the account. These returned checks are often marked "NSF" (Not Sufficient Funds).

1.10 a) Card security code

The card security code (CSC) is a three or four-digit number on the back of a credit card, to the right of the signature box.

1.11 a) Check

A check is a written, dated, and signed document that directs a bank to pay a specific sum of money to the bearer.

1.12 d) Plan

The plan section of a SOAP note is where the practitioner documents the treatment plan for the patient. This section typically includes the proposed treatment and may also include medication options, discharge instructions, follow-up instructions, and referrals.

1.13 c) 45–50

Current guidelines recommend starting colorectal cancer screening at the age of 45–50.

1.14 c) Every 1 year

The risk of breast cancer increases as women get older. The American Cancer Society (ACS) recommends annual mammograms for women aged 45–54, and the American College of Radiology recommends annual mammograms for all women over 40.

Content Area 2

Checking-In Patients

There are 14 questions in this content area.

2.1 Which federal law requires emergency departments to stabilize and treat anyone, regardless of their insurance status or ability to pay?
   a) Emergency Medical Treatment and Labor Act (EMTALA)
   b) Health Insurance Portability and Accountability Act (HIPAA)
   c) Occupational Safety and Health Act (OSHA)
   d) Patient Protection and Affordable Care Act (ACA)

2.2 A medical assistant prints out a patient's demographic information so the patient can review it for errors. Once the patient has reviewed the information, what should the medical assistant do with it?
   a) Dispose of it by shredding
   b) Give it to the doctor
   c) Give it to the patient to take home
   d) Put it in the patient's file

Answers on page 19

2.3 A patient has a health insurance plan with a $25 copay for doctor visits. She goes to the doctor three times in one month. What is the total amount she will pay in copays for the month?
  a) $50
  b) $25
  c) $0
  d) $75

2.4 A patient has a health insurance plan that pays 50% of allowed charges for out-of-network doctor visits. The patient visits an out-of-network doctor and the bill comes to $100. The health insurance allows only a $50 charge for the visit. How much would the patient have to pay out of pocket for the visit?
  a) $25
  b) $50
  c) $75
  d) $100

2.5 An arrangement where the patient pays for part of their medical expenses and the insurer pays for the rest is called a:
  a) co-pay
  b) deductible
  c) modifier
  d) premium

2.6 Medicare Part B pays for _____ of approved charges.
  a) 50%
  b) 60%
  c) 70%
  d) 80%

2.7 The date an insurance policy begins is known as the _____ date.
  a) coverage
  b) disclosure
  c) effective
  d) embarkation

Answers on page 19

2.8 What does 1EG4-TE5-MK72 on this card represent?

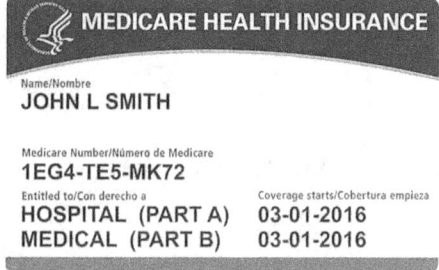

a) Insurance policy number
b) Medicare Beneficiary Identifier
c) Medicare's phone number
d) Social Security Number

2.9 What is the difference between copays and coinsurance?
a) Copays apply to medications, while coinsurance covers medical services
b) Copays are charged after the deductible is met, while coinsurance applies before the deductible is met
c) Copays are fixed costs, while coinsurance is percentage-based
d) Copays are paid at the end of the year, while coinsurance is paid at the time of service

2.10 An unconscious man is brought into an emergency ward. A medical assistant tries using his driver's license to find him in the hospital database. The date of birth on the license reads 07/12/1987 but the date the assistant enters into the computer is 07/21/1987. What type of error is this?
a) Double entry
b) Omission
c) Transposition
d) Truncation

2.11 Which of these should be written on a patient's wristband?
a) Bay number
b) Bed number
c) Medical record number
d) Room number

Answers on page 19

2.12 On this patient's wristband, what does 12-19-2016 mean?

Michelle Teoh
SEX F   TYPE A+
DR PAUL JOHNSON
ADM 12-19-2016

a) Admission date
b) Date of birth
c) Date of death
d) Date the patient started taking medication

2.13 Once patient registration is complete, the patient should receive a copy of which of the following?
a) A list of CLIA-waived tests
b) HIPAA Notice of Privacy Practices
c) The hospital's mission statement
d) Vaccine information statement

2.14 Which of these documents is suitable as legal photo identification?
a) Company-issued employee ID card
b) Credit card
c) Driver's license
d) Student ID card

Answers on page 20

ANSWERS

2.1 a) Emergency Medical Treatment and Labor Act (EMTALA)

The Emergency Medical Treatment and Active Labor Act requires hospital emergency departments to examine and treat anyone seeking treatment for a medical condition regardless of citizenship, legal status, or ability to pay.

2.2 a) Dispose of it by shredding

Once a patient has reviewed their printed demographic information for errors, the medical assistant should dispose of it by shredding. This ensures the patient's information remains confidential, thereby complying with privacy regulations.

2.3 d) $75

3 visits × $25/visit = $75.

2.4 c) $75

The health plan would pay 50% of the $50 allowed charge, which is $25. The patient would have to pay the other $75.

2.5 a) co-pay

A co-pay is an amount a patient has to pay every time they seek medical care. For example, a patient may need to pay $15 every time they see their doctor. Their insurance company pays for the rest.

2.6 d) 80%

Medicare Part B covers 80% of approved charges. This means the patient pays the remaining 20%.

2.7 c) effective

The effective date is the date an insurance policy officially becomes active.

2.8 b) Medicare Beneficiary Identifier

A Medicare Beneficiary Identifier (MBI) is a random string of letters and numbers assigned to every person with Medicare.

2.9 c) Copays are fixed costs, while coinsurance is percentage-based

Copays are a set fee the patient pays upfront for certain services. For example, if a doctor's visit has a $20 copay and the visit costs $200, the patient would pay $20 and the insurance company would pay the remaining $180.

Coinsurance is like copays except it works by percentage. If a patient has a 30% coinsurance policy, he must pay 30% of his medical bills and his insurance company will pay the remaining 70%. Note that coinsurance only comes into effect once the patient has met their deductible. If the patient hasn't met the deductible yet, he would have to pay the full bill upfront.

2.10 c) Transposition

A transpositional error is when two digits are accidentally swapped. In this case, the assistant swapped the digits 1 and 2 in the day part of the date, entering 07/21/1987 instead of 07/12/1987.

2.11 c) Medical record number

A medical record number is unique to each patient within a healthcare facility. It allows for quick and accurate identification, reducing the risk of confusion with other patients.

Room and bay numbers are unacceptable because they are not unique: multiple patients may share the same room or bay.

Bed number is unacceptable because if a patient changes bed, the number on the wristband would then be wrong.

2.12 a) Admission date

ADM is an abbreviation for "admission".

2.13 b) HIPAA Notice of Privacy Practices

New patients registering at a hospital or clinic must receive a copy of the HIPAA Notice of Privacy Practices. This document tells the patient how the hospital or clinic will use their health information.

Vaccine information statements (VIS) are given before a patient receives a vaccine.

2.14 c) Driver's license

For photo identification to be legal, it must be a government-issued ID. This includes a driver's license, passport, green card, permanent resident card, and military ID.

Content Area 3

Rooming Patients

There are 24 questions in this content area.

3.1 Which of these is a sign that a patient is stressed?
   a) Willingness to do as you ask
   b) Crying
   c) Constricted pupils
   d) Eye contact

3.2 When you suspect someone might be trans-identified, how do you know which pronoun to use?
   a) Ask a family member of the person
   b) Ask the person what pronouns they prefer
   c) Decide based on a person's appearance
   d) Use the pronoun of the person's biological gender

3.3 What does the PHQ-9 measure?
   a) Degree of cognitive impairment
   b) Depression severity
   c) Pain intensity
   d) Symptoms of drug abuse

Answers on page 27

3.4 What tool screens for anxiety?
- a) CAGE questionnaire
- b) GAD-7
- c) PHQ-9
- d) PSYRATS

3.5 You think a patient's name is John Smith but you are unsure. Which of these is the best question to confirm the patient's name?
- a) "Are you John Smith?"
- b) "I have to confirm your name. Can you confirm that your name is John Smith?"
- c) "Is your name the same as the name written here on this form?"
- d) "What is your name?"

3.6 How should a medical assistant prepare a patient for a punch biopsy?
- a) Anesthetize the site
- b) Clean the skin with a povidone-iodine solution
- c) Place the patient in the lithotomy position
- d) Put on sterile gloves

3.7 Which of these is found in a dressing pack?
- a) Mask
- b) Scalpel
- c) Scissors
- d) Swabs

3.8 A patient says he has burned his leg. What would be an appropriate question to screen for a medical emergency?
- a) "Are you able to drive a car?"
- b) "Are you married?"
- c) "Are you taking any medications?"
- d) "How did the burn happen?"

Answers on page 27

3.9 The CAGE questionnaire is used to help diagnose which health problem?
   a) Alcoholism
   b) Post-natal depression
   c) Schizophrenia
   d) Sleeping disorders

3.10 Which of these would you place in the "S" section when using SOAP charting?
   a) Patient's description of symptoms
   b) Physician's diagnosis
   c) Physician's examination
   d) Test results

3.11 Which of these questions is relevant when asking a patient about their current medications?
   a) "Does your insurance cover the cost of your medications?"
   b) "How often do you take your medication?"
   c) "What medications have you used in the past?"
   d) "Where do you buy your medications?"

3.12 What is the purpose of medication reconciliation?
   a) To ensure the patient understands how to take their medication
   b) To identify medication errors
   c) To reduce the workload of the pharmacy
   d) To update the patient's medication list with new prescriptions

3.13 What is a relevant question to ask a patient when assessing their neurological system?
   a) "Do you experience dizziness?"
   b) "Do you have a cough?"
   c) "Do you have any rashes?"
   d) "Do you have joint pain?"

Answers on page 28

3.14 Which of these questions is pertinent to taking a patient's past medical history?
 a) "Do any of your family members have health problems?"
 b) "Do you have any dietary restrictions?"
 c) "Have you ever been hospitalized?"
 d) "How often do you drink alcohol?"

3.15 What is the best question to determine a patient's chief complaint?
 a) "Do you have any allergies?"
 b) "Have you had any recent illnesses?"
 c) "What were you doing before you came here?"
 d) "What brings you here today?"

3.16 What is a relevant question to ask a patient when assessing their endocrine system?
 a) "Do you have chest pain?"
 b) "Do you sweat excessively?"
 c) "Have you ever coughed up blood?"
 d) "Have you had any genital discharge?"

3.17 What is the purpose of a health screening questionnaire?
 a) To assess the patient's mental health needs
 b) To ensure patients receive only the treatment they need
 c) To ensure the patient's insurance company will pay for the treatment
 d) To identify health problems before the patient is admitted

3.18 A patient looks dishevelled. His speech is disorganized; he jumps from topic to topic, making it difficult to follow what he is saying. He says he has started hearing voices that comment on his actions. What problem does the patient most likely have?
 a) Bipolar disorder
 b) Cushing's syndrome
 c) Hypothyroidism
 d) Schizophrenia

Answers on page 28

3.19 In healthcare, what does the abbreviation H&P mean?
   a) Health and psychology
   b) Heart rate and pressure
   c) History and physical
   d) Hospital and pharmaceutical

3.20 Which patient position is used to examine the abdomen?
   a) Prone
   b) Sims
   c) Sitting
   d) Supine

3.21 Which position is this patient in?

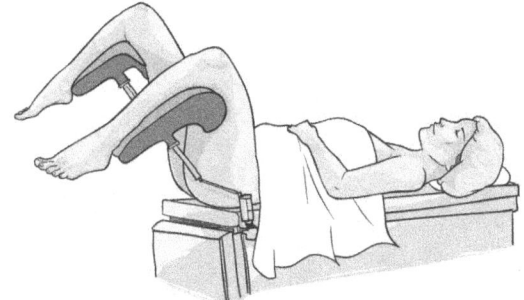

   a) Fowler
   b) Knee-chest
   c) Lithotomy
   d) Sim's

Answers on page 28

3.22 Which position is this patient in?

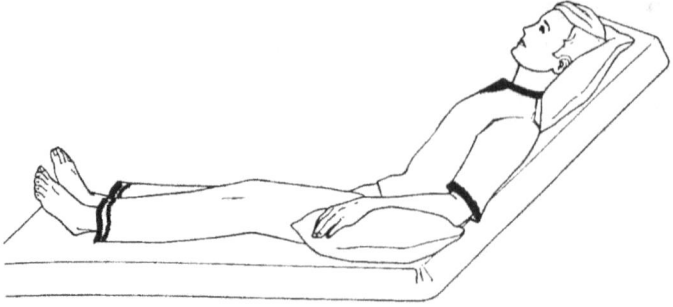

a) Fowler's
b) Lithotomy
c) Sim's
d) Trendenlenburg

3.23 A patient states on his health screening questionnaire that he is taking warfarin, aspirin, and ibuprofen. These medications increase the patient's risk of:
a) bleeding
b) cardiac arrest
c) diabetes
d) stroke

3.24 What does a MAR chart show?
a) A patient's daily activities and appointments
b) A patient's daily meal plans and nutrition intake
c) The drugs that have been administered to a patient
d) The exercises in a patient's physical therapy regimen

Answers on page 29

ANSWERS

3.1 b) Crying

Patients may cry when scared or stressed.

"Constricted pupils" is incorrect because stress causes pupils to dilate, not constrict.

3.2 b) Ask the person what pronouns they prefer

Because you can't assume gender identity from appearance or biology, the respectful approach is to ask the person directly.

3.3 b) Depression severity

The PHQ-9 (Patient Health Questionnaire-9) is a tool to measure the severity of depression.

3.4 b) GAD-7

The Generalized Anxiety Disorder 7 (GAD-7) is a self-reported questionnaire for screening and severity measuring of generalized anxiety disorder (GAD).

3.5 d) "What is your name?"

Asking the patient to say his name is better than asking him to respond "yes" or "no". The patient may have hearing or cognitive problems, meaning he would respond "yes" to any question.

3.6 b) Clean the skin with a povidone-iodine solution

Cleaning the skin before a punch biopsy is important to prevent infection.

Anesthetizing the site is performed by the physician, not a medical assistant.

The lithotomy position (feet in stirrups) is unnecessary for a punch biopsy.

Putting on sterile gloves would be the responsibility of the physician performing the biopsy.

3.7 d) Swabs

Dressing packs include swabs for cleaning and prepping wounds.

3.8 d) "How did the burn happen?"

"How did the burn happen?" would tell you the cause of the burn, which can help you determine if it is a medical emergency.

3.9 a) Alcoholism

The CAGE questionnaire is a 4-question screening tool that helps diagnose alcoholism.

3.10 a) Patient's description of symptoms

The S in SOAP stands for "subjective symptoms". This section records the patient's descriptions of their symptoms as expressed in their own words

3.11 b) "How often do you take your medication?"

When reviewing a patient's medications, information to ask for may include:

- the name of the medication
- the dosage and frequency
- the way the patient takes the medication
- the reason the patient is taking it
- how they have been long taking it
- does the patient feel it is working
- is the patient experiencing any side effects

3.12 b) To identify medication errors

Medication reconciliation is comparing the medications a patient should be taking to the medications they actually are taking. The process helps to identify any discrepancies, interactions, or errors.

3.13 a) "Do you experience dizziness?"

Dizziness is a common symptom of neurological problems. Parkinson's disease and multiple sclerosis are two examples of neurological disorders that cause dizziness.

3.14 c) "Have you ever been hospitalized?"

Past medical history is anything that happened to the patient's health before the present illness. It includes injuries, operations, significant illnesses, and hospitalizations.

3.15 d) "What brings you here today?"

Asking "What brings you here today?" encourages the patient to explain their main reason for seeking medical attention.

3.16 b) "Do you sweat excessively?"

Excessive sweating is a symptom of hyperthyroidism, an endocrine disorder.

3.17 d) To identify health problems before the patient is admitted

A health screening questionnaire gathers information about a patient's health status and history. This helps healthcare providers identify any existing health problems or risk factors that may need to be considered during the patient's stay in the hospital.

3.18 d) Schizophrenia

The patient exhibits two key symptoms of schizophrenia: disorganized speech (jumping from topic to topic) and auditory hallucinations (hearing voices).

3.19 c) History and physical

The H&P, or History and Physical, is an initial evaluation of the patient. "History" is the patient's medical history and "Physical" is a physical examination of the patient.

3.20 d) Supine

The supine position – lying on the back – is used to examine the head, chest, abdomen, and extremities.

3.21 c) Lithotomy

The patient in the image is in the lithotomy position. In the lithotomy position, the patient lies on their back with their legs up in stirrups. This position is used for gynecological procedures and childbirth.

3.22 a) Fowler's

Fowler's position is also known as the sitting position. In this position, the patient sits on a bed with their legs straight or slightly bent. The back is at an angle of 45–60 degrees.

3.23 a) bleeding

All three medications reduce the clotting ability of blood. Warfarin is an anticoagulant and aspirin and ibuprofen both inhibit platelet aggregation. When taken together, these medications significantly increase the risk of bleeding.

3.24 c) The drugs that have been administered to a patient

A medication administration record (MAR) chart records the drugs a patient has received while in care.

Content Area 4

Collecting Patient Vitals

There are 39 questions in this content area.

4.1 What is the medical term for high blood pressure?
   a) Hyperalbuminemia
   b) Hyperglycemia
   c) Hyperplasia
   d) Hypertension

4.2 A high-pitched, wheezing sound caused by disrupted airflow is called:
   a) asthma
   b) diphtheria
   c) epistaxis
   d) stridor

4.3 What is the medical term for low levels of oxygen in the blood?
   a) Hematemesis
   b) Hemorrhage
   c) Hypoxemia
   d) Paroxysmal

Answers on page 38

4.4 What is the medical term for fever?
  a) Hypertension
  b) Hypothermia
  c) Pyrexia
  d) Tachypnea

4.5 What is the medical term for difficulty breathing when lying down?
  a) Dysphonia
  b) Dyspnea
  c) Hemothorax
  d) Orthopnea

4.6 What is the medical term for rapid breathing?
  a) Eupepsia
  b) Hyperkalemia
  c) Peritonitis
  d) Tachypnea

4.7 What is the medical term for shortness of breath?
  a) Anosmia
  b) Ascites
  c) Dyspnea
  d) Phlebitis

4.8 Tachycardia is defined as a heart rate of how many beats per minute?
  a) 40–60 bpm
  b) 60–80 bpm
  c) 80–100 bpm
  d) >100 bpm

4.9 What is the term for a heartbeat of fewer than 60 beats per minute?
  a) Bradycardia
  b) Epicardia
  c) Myocardia
  d) Tachycardia

Answers on page 38

4.10 A patient is 2 meters tall and weighs 100 kg. Calculate the patient's body mass index.
   a) 15
   b) 20
   c) 25
   d) 40

4.11 The normal oxygen saturation in blood is _____ or higher.
   a) 50%
   b) 66%
   c) 90%
   d) 95%

4.12 Which of these patients should be taken to a doctor immediately?
   a) A patient with itchy eyes, sneezing, and a runny nose
   b) A patient with an itchy rash on their arm after trying a new lotion
   c) A patient with chest discomfort and a blood pressure of 220/120
   d) A patient with cough, chills, and a temperature of 100.4°F (38.0°C)

4.13 What does a sphygmomanometer measure?
   a) Blood pressure
   b) Body temperature
   c) Motor reflexes
   d) The density of liquids

4.14 Which medical term means a normal body temperature?
   a) Afebrile
   b) Febrile
   c) Hyperpyrexic
   d) Hypopyrexic

Answers on page 39

4.15 Where is an axillary temperature taken?
   a) Anus
   b) Armpit
   c) Ear
   d) Forehead

4.16 What pulse is located on the top of the foot?
   a) Carotid
   b) Dorsalis pedis
   c) Femoral
   d) Popliteal

4.17 What is the normal range for diastolic blood pressure in adults?
   a) 40–69 mmHg
   b) 60–79 mmHg
   c) 90–119 mmHg
   d) 120–139 mmHg

4.18 The normal respiratory rate for adults is _____ breaths per minute.
   a) 4–12
   b) 12–20
   c) 20–28
   d) 28–36

4.19 A patient's blood pressure is 150/100. What is the patient's pulse pressure?
   a) 1.5
   b) 50
   c) 100
   d) 150

4.20 Pulse oximeters are generally attached to which body part?
   a) Earlobe
   b) Finger
   c) Forehead
   d) Wrist

Answers on page 39

4.21 Where is the apical pulse found?
- a) Behind the knee
- b) On the throat
- c) On the wrist
- d) Over the heart

4.22 Where is the temporal pulse point located?
- a) Armpit
- b) Forehead
- c) Mouth
- d) Rectum

4.23 Which of these factors can interfere with the accuracy of pulse oximetry readings?
- a) Blood type
- b) Fingernail polish
- c) High blood pressure
- d) The contents of the patient's previous meal

4.24 What is the normal range for systolic blood pressure in adults?
- a) 40–69 mm Hg
- b) 60–79 mm Hg
- c) 90–119 mm Hg
- d) 120–139 mm Hg

4.25 Where is a tympanic temperature taken?
- a) Ear
- b) Forehead
- c) Mouth
- d) Rectum

4.26 A normal resting heart rate for adults is _____ beats per minute.
- a) 40 to 80
- b) 60 to 100
- c) 80 to 120
- d) 100 to 140

Answers on page 40

4.27 Which pulse is used to measure blood pressure when the brachial pulse is inaccessible?
   a) Dorsalis pedis
   b) Femoral
   c) Popliteal
   d) Posterior tibial

4.28 What is the most accurate place to measure a person's body temperature?
   a) Anus
   b) Armpit
   c) Ears
   d) Mouth

4.29 What non-invasive test measures blood oxygen levels?
   a) Bioimpedance analysis
   b) Blood gas analysis
   c) Capnography
   d) Pulse oximetry

4.30 What is normal body temperature?
   a) 21°C
   b) 32°C
   c) 37°C
   d) 100°C

4.31 A patient and his wheelchair together weigh 100 kg. The wheelchair alone weighs 20 kg. How much does the patient weigh?
   a) 80 kg
   b) 100 kg
   c) 120 kg
   d) 130 kg

Answers on page 40

4.32 Which artery in the wrist is used for measuring a person's pulse?
   a) Carotid
   b) Radial
   c) Temporal
   d) Ulnar

4.33 What is the BMI overweight range?
   a) 16–18.49
   b) 18.5–24.9
   c) 25–29.99
   d) 30–34.99

4.34 Which of these temperatures is the highest?
   a) Axillary
   b) Oral
   c) Rectal
   d) Temporal

4.35 What pulse is located in the middle of the groin?
   a) Carotid
   b) Dorsalis pedis
   c) Femoral
   d) Popliteal

4.36 What is the abbreviation for the amount of oxygen in the blood as a percentage of the maximum the blood could carry?
   a) BO_2
   b) $HgbO_2$
   c) $O_2\%$
   d) SpO_2

4.37 Before measuring a patient's weight:
   a) ask the patient to put on their shoes
   b) calibrate the scale by standing on it
   c) empty any urinary catheter bags
   d) put on a gown and sterile gloves

Answers on page 41

4.38 What type of thermometer can measure oral, axillary, and rectal temperatures?
   a) Digital
   b) Laboratory
   c) Temporal artery
   d) Tympanic

4.39 Which position is used to measure a patient's vital signs?
   a) Fowler's
   b) Lithotomy
   c) Prone
   d) Sitting

Answers on page 41

ANSWERS

4.1 d) Hypertension

Hypertension is the medical term for high blood pressure. The word is from hyper (meaning "high") and tension (meaning "pressure").

Hyperalbuminemia is an abnormally high level of albumin in the blood.

Hyperglycemia is abnormally high blood sugar levels.

Hyperplasia is increased cell production in a tissue or organ.

4.2 d) stridor

Stridor is noisy breathing that occurs due to obstructed air flow through a narrowed airway.

4.3 c) Hypoxemia

Hypoxemia is the term for a below-normal level of oxygen in the blood. The word is derived from *hypo* (low) + *oxy* (oxygen) + *emia* (blood).

4.4 c) Pyrexia

Pyrexia is the medical term for fever.

Option a, hypertension, is high blood pressure.

Option b, hypothermia, is a dangerously low body temperature, below 95°F.

Option d, tachypnea, is rapid breathing.

4.5 d) Orthopnea

Orthopnea is shortness of breath or difficulty breathing when lying down. It comes from the Greek words "ortho," which means straight or vertical, and "pnea," which means to breathe.

4.6 d) Tachypnea

Tachypnea is a respiratory rate greater than normal. The word comes from tachy (fast) + pnea (breathing).

Eupepsia means normal digestion.

Hyperkalemia means high blood potassium.

Peritonitis is inflammation of the peritoneum.

4.7 c) Dyspnea

Dyspnea means difficulty breathing. The word comes from *dys-*, meaning "bad", and *pnea*, meaning "breathing".

Anosmia is the inability to smell.

Ascites is the build of fluid in the abdomen.

Phlebitis means inflammation of a vein.

4.8 d) >100 bpm

Tachycardia is a heart rate of over 100 beats a minute. *Tachy-* means "fast" and *-cardia* means "heart".

4.9 a) Bradycardia

Bradycardia means a slow heartbeat. The word bradycardia is from *brady* (meaning "slow") and *cardia* (meaning "heart").

Option b, the epicardium (plural: epicardia), is the outer layer of the heart.

Option c, the myocardium (plural: myocardia), is the heart's muscular tissue.

Option d, tachycardia, is a fast heart rate, over 100 beats a minute.

4.10 c) 25

The equation for body mass index is:

$$\text{body mass index} = \frac{\text{weight (in kg)}}{\text{height (in meters)}^2}$$

Inserting the values from the question into the equation:

$$\text{body mass index} = \frac{100}{2^2}$$

$$= \frac{100}{4}$$

$$= 25$$

4.11 d) 95%

Oxygen saturation (SpO2) is the percentage of hemoglobin carrying oxygen. The normal oxygen saturation (SpO2) is 95% or higher.

4.12 c) A patient with chest discomfort and a blood pressure of 220/120

A blood pressure of 220/120 is critically high. This, along with the patient's chest discomfort, could indicate a serious medical condition, such as a heart attack or stroke. This patient requires immediate medical attention.

4.13 a) Blood pressure

A sphygmomanometer, also known as a blood pressure monitor, measures blood pressure. It consists of an inflatable cuff which is wrapped around the arm.

4.14 a) Afebrile

Febrile means feverish. Adding the prefix *a-* (meaning "without" or "not") to "febrile" creates "afebrile", a term meaning not feverish.

4.15 b) Armpit

Axillary means the armpit.

4.16 b) Dorsalis pedis

The dorsalis pedis artery is located on the upper surface of the foot.

4.17 b) 60–79 mmHg

Normal diastolic pressure is between 60 and 79 mmHg.

4.18 b) 12–20

The normal respiration rate for an adult at rest ranges from 12 to 20 breaths per minute.

4.19 b) 50

Pulse pressure is the difference between systolic and diastolic blood pressure. In the question, the systolic pressure is 150 and the diastolic pressure is 100. Therefore the pulse pressure is:

$$150 - 100 = 50$$

4.20 b) Finger

Pulse oximeters are generally attached to a finger, although they can also be attached to the forehead, nose, foot, ears or toes.

4.21 d) Over the heart

The apical pulse is found over the apex of the heart.

4.22 b) Forehead

The temporal artery is a major artery of the head that runs laterally across the forehead and down the side of the neck. It is the place where forehead temperature is taken from.

For reference, here are the other pulse points:

- Carotid – throat
- Brachial – inside the elbow
- Radial – wrist
- Femoral – groin
- Popliteal – back of the knee
- Posterior tibial – inside ankle
- Dorsalis Pedis – top of foot

4.23 b) Fingernail polish

Dark nail polish can block the light signals pulse oximeters use to measure blood oxygen levels.

4.24 c) 90–119 mm Hg

Normal systolic pressure is between 90 and 119 mm Hg.

4.25 a) Ear

The word "tympanic" means the eardrum. A tympanic temperature is taken by inserting a thermometer into the auditory canal, where it comes into close contact with the eardrum.

4.26 b) 60 to 100

A normal resting heart rate for adults ranges from 60 to 100 beats per minute.

4.27 c) Popliteal

The popliteal pulse is located at the back of the knee and is detected most easily when the knee is slightly flexed. This site can be used to measure blood pressure when the brachial pulse is inaccessible.

4.28 a) Anus

The anus provides the most accurate measurement of body temperature because fewer factors can affect the results.

4.29 d) Pulse oximetry

Pulse oximetry is a non-invasive test that measures blood oxygen levels. The test sends light beams through the finger into a detector on the other side. The pulse oximeter estimates blood oxygen levels by measuring how much light the blood absorbs.

Bioimpedance analysis does not measure blood oxygen levels. It estimates body composition, in particular body fat and muscle mass.

Blood gas analysis measures various blood components, including oxygen levels. However, it requires drawing blood, which makes it an invasive test.

Capnography measures carbon dioxide, not oxygen.

4.30 c) 37°C

Normal human body temperature is around 37 degrees Celsius (98.6 degrees Fahrenheit).

4.31 a) 80 kg

To find the patient's weight, subtract the weight of the wheelchair from the combined weight of the wheelchair and patient:

$$100 \text{ kg} - 20 \text{ kg} = 80 \text{ kg}$$

4.32 b) Radial

The most common site for measuring the pulse is the radial artery on the inner wrist, just below the thumb. The radial pulse is taken by placing two fingertips on the wrist.

The carotid artery is also used for measuring pulse but this artery is located in the neck, not the wrist.

4.33 **c) 25–29.99**

People with a BMI of 25 to 29.99 are considered overweight.

18.49 and below is the underweight range.

18.5–24.9 is the normal range.

30.0 and above is the obese range.

4.34 **c) Rectal**

Of the temperatures listed, rectal temperature is considered the highest. Rectal temperature is the most accurate reflection of the body's core temperature.

Armpit (axillary) and forehead (temporal) temperature is usually around 1°C (1.8°F) lower than rectal temperature.

Oral temperature is usually around 0.5 °C (0.9°F) lower than rectal temperature.

4.35 **c) Femoral**

The femoral pulse is in the middle of the groin.

4.36 **d) SpO_2**

SpO2 stands for saturation of peripheral oxygen. It is a measure of the amount of oxygen in the blood.

4.37 **c) empty any urinary catheter bags**

It is important to empty urinary catheter bags before weighing a patient. This is because the weight of the urine can affect the accuracy of the reading.

Option a, asking the patient to wear shoes during weighing, is unnecessary. In fact, ideally, the patient should not be wearing shoes. The exception is if the patient was wearing shoes in previous measurements, in which case, the patient should wear shoes for all future weighings to ensure consistency across the results.

Option b, calibrating the scale by standing on it, is not how scales are calibrated. Scales are typically calibrated using special calibration weights.

Option d, putting on a gown and gloves, is unnecessary unless there are specific hygiene protocols.

4.38 **a) Digital**

The correct answer is digital thermometers. Most digital thermometers can be used for oral, axillary, and rectal measurements.

Option b, laboratory, is incorrect because laboratory thermometers are used in laboratories, not for measuring human body temperature.

Option c, temporal artery, is incorrect because temporal artery thermometers are used for measuring forehead temperature.

Option d, tympanic, is incorrect because tympanic thermometers only measure ear temperature. "Tympanic" refers to the tympanic membrane, another name for the ear drum.

4.39 **d) Sitting**

Generally, the sitting position is used to measure heart rate, temperature, blood pressure, and other vital signs. The supine position (lying flat on the back, facing upwards) and standing position may also be used.

Content Area 5

Performing Point of Care Orders

There are 100 questions in this content area.

5.1 Which vein should be tried first when choosing a draw site?
   a) Basilic
   b) Cephalic
   c) Median antibrachial
   d) Median cubital

Answers on page 63

5.2 Which letter is pointing to the median cubital vein?

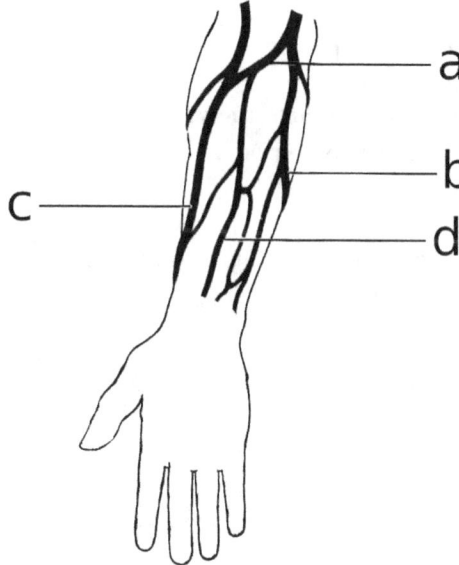

   a) a
   b) b
   c) c
   d) d

5.3 Why must the phlebotomist clean the patient's skin before performing a venipuncture?
   a) To increase blood flow to the area
   b) To make the veins more prominent
   c) To remove microorganisms
   d) To remove oil and sweat

5.4 Petechiae appear when a phlebotomist applies a tourniquet to a patient's arm. What should the phlebotomist do?
   a) Call a nurse
   b) Cancel the draw
   c) Continue with the draw
   d) Try the other arm

Answers on page 63

5.5 What might happen if an angle of 8 degrees is used when performing venipuncture?
   a) A deep hematoma may form
   b) The needle may enter above the vein
   c) The needle may go completely through the vein
   d) The needle may go through the posterior wall of the vein

5.6 During venipuncture, what is the longest time a tourniquet should remain on the patient's arm?
   a) 1 minute
   b) 3 minutes
   c) 5 minutes
   d) 7 minutes

5.7 A phlebotomist is collecting blood from the vein of a 14-month-old baby when the blood stops flowing. Which of these actions should the phlebotomist take to try to continue the draw?
   a) Give the baby something sweet to eat
   b) Release the tourniquet
   c) Try a new tube
   d) Try to collect blood from the baby's heel instead

5.8 Repeated phlebotomy procedures in the same area can cause:
   a) petechiae
   b) scarring
   c) thrombosis
   d) varicose veins

5.9 Which of these needles has the largest diameter?
   a) 18-gauge
   b) 19-gauge
   c) 20-gauge
   d) 21-gauge

Answers on page 64

5.10 A winged infusion set is also called a _____ needle.
   a) Milliner's
   b) butterfly
   c) straight
   d) universal

5.11 Which of these analytes is photosensitive?
   a) Albumin
   b) Bilirubin
   c) Iron
   d) Phosphate

5.12 Which of these conditions can be monitored using pulse oximetry?
   a) COPD
   b) Diabetes
   c) Hypertension
   d) Hypothyroidism

5.13 What is otitis?
   a) An abnormal discharge from the nose
   b) An eye infection
   c) Ear inflammation
   d) Inflammation of the sinuses

5.14 What is tinnitus?
   a) A false sense of motion or spinning
   b) A ringing sound in the ears
   c) A voice disorder
   d) Hearing loss that occurs with old age

5.15 What is another word for myopia?
   a) Astigmatism
   b) Farsightedness
   c) Nearsightedness
   d) Strabismus

Answers on page 64

5.16 What time of day does urine contain the highest concentration of human chorionic gonadotropin?
   a) Morning
   b) Afternoon
   c) Evening
   d) Night

5.17 Where is the preferred injection site for the PPD test?
   a) Arm
   b) Hand
   c) Leg
   d) Shoulder

5.18 Tubersol and Aplisol are antigens used for which test?
   a) Flu test
   b) Hemoglobin test
   c) PPD test
   d) Strep test

5.19 A positive PPD test is shown by:
   a) edema
   b) erythema
   c) fever
   d) induration

5.20 The PPD test detects which disease?
   a) Bronchitis
   b) Influenza
   c) Pneumonia
   d) Tuberculosis

5.21 Which area is swabbed to obtain a throat culture?
   a) Larynx
   b) Oral mucosa
   c) Pharynx
   d) Trachea

Answers on page 65

5.22 From where is a specimen for a rapid strep test obtained?
   a) Ear canal
   b) Nasopharynx
   c) Nose
   d) Throat

5.23 Pregnancy test strips detect the presence of which hormone?
   a) Adrenocorticotropic hormone
   b) Estrogen
   c) Human chorionic gonadotropin
   d) Progesterone

5.24 Urine is applied to a pregnancy strip. After several minutes, the strip shows no lines. This means the result is:
   a) inconclusive
   b) invalid
   c) negative
   d) positive

5.25 How far into the nasal cavity must a swab be inserted to reach the nasopharynx?
   a) 3–4 cm
   b) 5–6 cm
   c) 7–8 cm
   d) 9–10 cm

5.26 Which urine collection technique collects urine by inserting a sterile needle into the patient's bladder through the abdominal wall?
   a) Biopsy
   b) Necropsy
   c) Suprapubic aspiration
   d) Urinary catheter

Answers on page 65

5.27 What is the initial screening test for Cushing syndrome?
   a) C-reactive protein test
   b) Comprehensive metabolic panel
   c) Erythrocyte sedimentation rate
   d) Urinary free cortisol test

5.28 Midstream urine samples are most often used for:
   a) culture and susceptibility
   b) mononucleosis testing
   c) pregnancy testing
   d) routine urinalysis

5.29 Which test measures a patient's average blood glucose level over the last two to three months?
   a) Blood insulin
   b) Glucose tolerance test
   c) HbA1c
   d) Random blood glucose test

5.30 How many acceptable attempts must be obtained when measuring a patient's peak flow rate?
   a) 1
   b) 3
   c) 2
   d) 4

5.31 What unit is the peak flow rate measured in?
   a) L/min
   b) liters
   c) mm
   d) seconds

5.32 How should a patient breathe into a peak flow meter?
   a) As fast and hard as possible
   b) Normally
   c) Slowly and gently
   d) With short, shallow breaths

Answers on page 66

5.33 In the peak flow zone system, which zone is a score of 50–80% of the patient's normal peak flow?
   a) Black
   b) Green
   c) Red
   d) Yellow

5.34 The peak flow test is used to diagnose and monitor:
   a) angina
   b) asthma
   c) cystitis
   d) hypertension

5.35 Why are finger punctures made at right angles to fingerprint striations?
   a) To facilitate blood sample collection
   b) To prevent excessive bleeding
   c) To prevent scar formation
   d) To reduce pain

5.36 Which term means the presence of glucose in the blood?
   a) Glycemia
   b) Glycogenolysis
   c) Glycolysis
   d) Glycosuria

5.37 Which fingers are used for finger puncture?
   a) Little finger and ring finger
   b) Little finger and thumb
   c) Middle finger and ring finger
   d) Ring finger and thumb

5.38 What do C and T mean on a pregnancy test?
   a) Clarity and time
   b) Color and temperature
   c) Consistency and translucency
   d) Control and test

Answers on page 67

5.39 What is the SI unit for reporting the result of urine glucose tests?
   a) mg/L
   b) mg/dL
   c) mmol/L
   d) mmol/dL

5.40 What color is the urine of patients with jaundice?
   a) Brownish-yellow
   b) Milky
   c) Red
   d) Straw-colored

5.41 What is the normal adult range for peak flow?
   a) 20–40 liters per minute
   b) 50–80 liters per minute
   c) 150–250 liters per minute
   d) 400–700 liters per minute

5.42 When performing ear irrigation, what temperature is recommended for the irrigating solution?
   a) Ice cold
   b) Room temperature
   c) Body temperature
   d) 50–52°C

5.43 How should a patient be positioned for ear irrigation?
   a) Lying down with the affected ear facing up
   b) Lying on the stomach with the head turned
   c) Sitting up with the head tilted slightly to the side
   d) Standing with the head tilted forward

5.44 What is a Noots tank?
   a) A cup to collect earwax during ear irrigation
   b) A device a person blows into for the peak flow test
   c) A portable oxygen tank for people with lung conditions
   d) A specialized container for hazardous waste disposal

Answers on page 67

5.45 What is a common side effect of ear irrigation?
   a) Blurred vision
   b) Dizziness
   c) Headache
   d) Rash

5.46 Which of these results should be reported to the doctor immediately?
   a) Blood glucose of 400 mg/dL
   b) Hemoglobin of 20 g/dL
   c) Peak flow score of 500 L/min
   d) Positive strep test

5.47 Otoscopes examine which part of the body?
   a) Ears
   b) Eyes
   c) Mouth
   d) Nose

5.48 Which of the following information should be included in an ECG report?
   a) The patient's insurance details
   b) The patient's weight
   c) The time of the recording
   d) Whether the patient was fasting

5.49 What does the Ishihara test detect?
   a) Color blindness
   b) Hearing loss
   c) Tuberculosis infection
   d) Visual acuity

5.50 In the Ishiwara test, how far should the plates be held away from the patient?
   a) 50 cm
   b) 75 cm
   c) 125 cm
   d) 150 cm

Answers on page 68

5.51 A patient has 20/30 vision. What does this mean?
  a) The patient can read letters from 20 feet away that most people can read from 30 feet away
  b) The patient can see at 30 feet what the average person could only see from 20 feet
  c) The patient correctly identified 20 out of 30 letters on a visual acuity test
  d) The patient has perfect vision in his left eye (20) and slightly worse vision in his right eye (30)

5.52 What is the medical term for nearsightedness?
  a) Astigmatism
  b) Hyperopia
  c) Myopia
  d) Presbyopia

5.53 How far should a patient stand from a Snellen eye chart?
  a) 5 feet
  b) 10 feet
  c) 15 feet
  d) 20 feet

5.54 Sound frequency is measured in:
  a) amplitude
  b) decibels
  c) hertz
  d) pascals

5.55 What variable is on the X-axis of audiograms?
  a) Frequency
  b) Hearing level
  c) Loudness
  d) Time

5.56 The loudness of sound is measured in:
  a) Joules
  b) Pascals
  c) decibels
  d) hertz

Answers on page 68

5.57 What is the term for hearing loss in only one ear?
- a) Directional
- b) Monaural
- c) Monophonic
- d) Unilateral

5.58 What is the normal range for hearing?
- a) 20–20,000 Hz
- b) 40–40,000 Hz
- c) 60–60,000 Hz
- d) 80–80,000 Hz

5.59 Which of these tools is used to assess hearing?
- a) Anoscope
- b) Percussion hammer
- c) Specimen collection system
- d) Tuning forks

5.60 Which part of a syringe has volume markings?
- a) Barrel
- b) Flange
- c) Needle
- d) Plunger

5.61 What view of the heart do leads II, III, and aVF of an electrocardiogram represent?
- a) Anterior
- b) Inferior
- c) Lateral
- d) Septal

5.62 In electrocardiography, what is the collective name for the aVR, aVL, and aVF leads?
- a) Alternating voltage leads
- b) Amplified voltage leads
- c) Augmented limb leads
- d) Depolarization-repolarization leads

Answers on page 69

5.63 Einthoven's law states:
   a) Lead I + Lead II = Lead III
   b) Lead I + Lead III = Lead II
   c) Lead I - Lead II = Lead III
   d) Lead I - Lead III = Lead II

5.64 Leads II, III, and aVF of an ECG are called the _____ leads.
   a) grounding
   b) inferior
   c) lateral
   d) limb

5.65 When preparing a patient for an electrocardiogram, where is the V3 electrode placed?
   a) Between the right shoulder and right wrist
   b) Fourth intercostal space to the left of the sternum
   c) Fourth intercostal space to the right of the sternum
   d) Midway between V2 and V4

5.66 Which three ECG electrodes form the Einthoven triangle?
   a) RA, LA and LL
   b) RA, LA and RL
   c) RA, LL and RL
   d) V1, V2 and V3

5.67 The Bazett formula corrects which interval?
   a) PR
   b) QT
   c) ST
   d) TP

5.68 When preparing a patient for an ECG, where should you place the V1 electrode?
   a) Arm
   b) Chest
   c) Foot
   d) Leg

Answers on page 69

5.69 Which electrodes are used for lead III in electrocardiography?
   a) LA and LL
   b) LA and RL
   c) RA and LL
   d) RA and RL

5.70 Which of these is a mistake when attaching ECG leads to a patient?
   a) Attaching the LA lead to the patient's left arm
   b) Attaching the LL lead to the patient's left leg
   c) Attaching the RL lead to the patient's right arm
   d) Attaching the V1 lead to the 4th intercostal space, right sternal edge

5.71 The special lead positions below help to diagnose which arrhythmia?

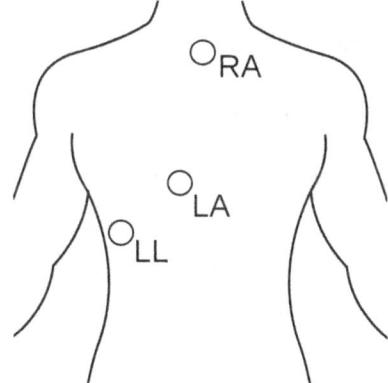

   a) Atrial flutter
   b) Bradycardia
   c) Ventricular fibrillation
   d) Ventricular tachycardia

Answers on page 70

5.72 Lead I of an ECG records differences between which electrodes?
 a) LA and RA
 b) LA and RL
 c) RA and LL
 d) RA and RL

5.73 For which condition might you need to increase the ECG paper speed?
 a) Adams–Stokes syndrome
 b) Bradycardia
 c) Bundle branch block
 d) Tachycardia

5.74 You are preparing a patient for an electrocardiogram but the patient's left lower leg is amputated. What should you do?
 a) Cancel the electrocardiogram
 b) Perform the electrocardiogram but without the LL and RL electrodes
 c) Perform the electrocardiogram but without the LL electrode
 d) Place the LL electrode above the patient's left knee instead

Answers on page 70

5.75 When setting up an ECG, where is the LA electrode placed?

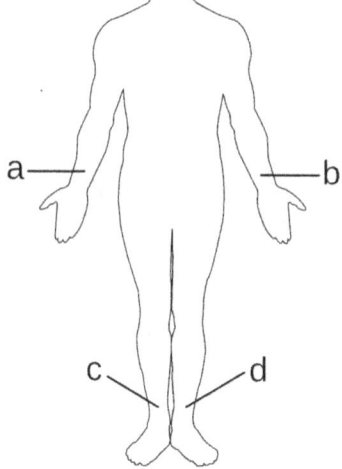

a) a
b) b
c) c
d) o

5.76 When applying chest leads for an electrocardiogram, where is V1 placed?
a) At the fifth intercostal space, left midclavicular line
b) At the fourth intercostal space, left sternal border
c) At the fourth intercostal space, right sternal border
d) Midway between V3 and V5

5.77 Why do ECG electrodes have tabs?
a) So the nurse can write notes on them
b) To attach alligator clips
c) To attach the electrode to the patient's skin
d) To prevent patient shocks

Answers on page 70

5.78 In electrocardiography, what does the letter A in aVL stand for?
   a) actual
   b) alternating
   c) amplitude
   d) augmented

5.79 A patient is undergoing a cardiac treadmill stress test when he starts showing signs of cardiac ischemia. What should you do?
   a) Ask the patient if he can keep going
   b) Slow down the treadmill to a more comfortable speed
   c) Speed up the treadmill
   d) Stop the test

5.80 Which of these statements about preparing a patient for an ECG is true?
   a) Alcohol wipes are used to clean the skin
   b) It is good practice to shave the patient's entire chest
   c) The patient must be fasting
   d) The patient should be sitting

5.81 When applying chest leads for an electrocardiogram, where is V2 placed?
   a) At the fifth intercostal space to the left of the midclavicular line
   b) At the fourth intercostal space to the left of the sternum
   c) At the fourth intercostal space to the right of the sternum
   d) Midway between V3 and V5

5.82 What is the normal paper speed for an ECG?
   a) 25 mm/second
   b) 50 mm/second
   c) 75 mm/second
   d) 100 mm/second

Answers on page 71

5.83 When performing an ECG, which of these steps comes first?
   a) Apply the limb electrodes
   b) Ask the patient to remove their clothing from the waist up
   c) Obtain the patient's consent
   d) Prepare the patient's skin for the application of the electrodes

5.84 Which ECG electrode is placed near the patient's right ankle?
   a) LA
   b) LL
   c) RA
   d) RL

5.85 The right leg (RL) electrode of the electrocardiogram is also known as:
   a) F
   b) N
   c) T
   d) V1

5.86 In the American Heart Association system of ECG lead color coding, what color is the neutral electrode?
   a) Black
   b) Green
   c) Red
   d) White

5.87 Why is paste or jelly applied to a patient before an ECG?
   a) To facilitate conductivity between the skin and the electrode
   b) To prevent the electrodes from overheating
   c) To reduce the risk of shocking the patient
   d) To reduce the risk of shocking the technician

Answers on page 71

5.88 What color is the RA electrode in the American Heart Association ECG lead color coding system?
   a) Black
   b) Green
   c) Red
   d) White

5.89 What view of the heart do leads I, aVL, V5, and V6 of an electrocardiogram represent?
   a) Anterior
   b) Inferior
   c) Lateral
   d) Septal

5.90 Which lead is best for measuring the QT interval?
   a) Lead I
   b) Lead II
   c) Lead III
   d) aVR

5.91 In electrocardiography, which lead is also called the augmented unipolar right arm lead?
   a) Lead I
   b) aVF
   c) aVL
   d) aVR

5.92 ECG leads I, II, and III are called the _____ limb leads.
   a) augmented
   b) bipolar
   c) positive
   d) unipolar

Answers on page 72

5.93 Which lead of an electrocardiogram is needed for a rhythm strip?
   a) I
   b) II
   c) III
   d) IV

5.94 Lead II of an ECG records differences between which electrodes?
   a) LA and LL
   b) LA and RA
   c) LA and RL
   d) RA and LL

5.95 Leads V1 to V6 are called the _____ leads.
   a) augmented
   b) cardiac
   c) chest
   d) limb

5.96 When applying chest leads for an electrocardiogram, where is V6 placed?
   a) Anywhere between the right shoulder and the wrist
   b) The fourth intercostal space to the left of the sternum
   c) The fourth intercostal space to the right of the sternum
   d) The midaxillary line at the same level as V4 and V5

5.97 How long is a normal standardization mark on an ECG tracing?
   a) 10 mm
   b) 15 mm
   c) 20 mm
   d) 25 mm

Answers on page 72

5.98 What artifact is in this ECG tracing?

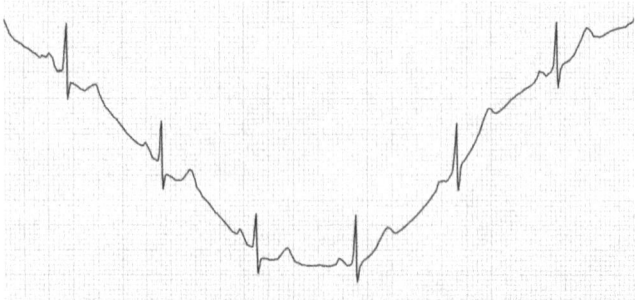

a) AC interference
b) Baseline wander
c) Loose lead
d) Muscle tremor

5.99 What artifact is in this ECG tracing?

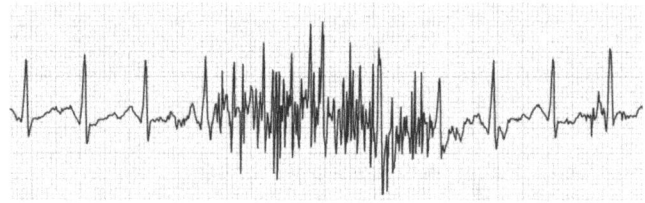

a) AC interference
b) CPR compression
c) Loose lead
d) Muscle tremor

5.100 What artifact is in this ECG tracing?

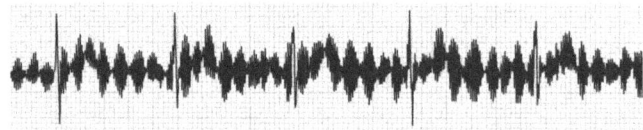

a) AC interference
b) Baseline wander
c) Loose lead
d) Muscle tremor

Answers on page 72

ANSWERS

5.1 d) Median cubital

The median cubital vein is preferred for venipuncture because it is large, easy to access, and unlikely to roll around.

5.2 a) a

The median cubital vein (or median basilic vein) is labelled "a" in the image. It is located inside the elbow. It is the first choice for venipuncture due to its size and accessibility.

The vein labelled "b" is the basilic vein. It is found on the medial (pinky side) aspect of the arm.

The vein labelled "c" is the cephalic vein. This vein runs along the lateral (thumb side) aspect of the arm.

The vein labelled "d" is the median vein. It runs along the center of the forearm.

Figure 1 shows the labelled veins.

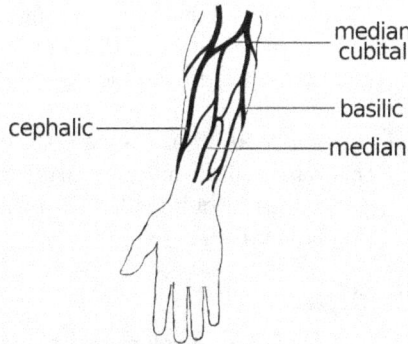

Figure 1: Diagram of the major veins in the arm, showing the cephalic, basilic, median cubital, and median veins.

5.3 c) To remove microorganisms

The purpose of cleaning the patient's skin is to remove microorganisms that could cause infection.

5.4 c) Continue with the draw

Petechiae (small red dots) after applying a tourniquet are not a cause for concern. They usually disappear after the procedure is completed.

Trying the other arm is unnecessary because the same reaction will likely occur.

5.5 b) The needle may enter above the vein

The ideal angle for insertion for venipuncture is 15 degrees. An angle less than 15 degrees may cause the needle to enter above the vein instead.

5.6 a) 1 minute

Tourniquets should be left on the patient's arm for less than a minute. Leaving the tourniquet on longer than a minute can affect test results due to hemoconcentration. It could also hurt the patient.

5.7 c) Try a new tube

The first step to try would be to replace the tube, as the tube may be defective. If this doesn't work, your next step should be to try to draw blood from the dorsal hand vein.

Option b, releasing the tourniquet, might cause the vein to collapse.

Option d, collecting blood from the heel,

is incorrect. The heel is not used to collect blood once the child begins to walk.

5.8 b) scarring

When venipunctures are repeated in the same area, scar tissue (sclerosing) can develop.

Option a, petechiae, are small red spots caused by bleeding disorders or from leaving a tourniquet on too long.

Option c, thrombosis, is not a typical result of venipuncture.

Option d, varicose veins, are not caused by venipuncture.

5.9 a) 18-gauge

Needle thickness is measured in gauges. The smaller the gauge number, the larger the diameter. For example, an 18-gauge needle is thicker than a 19-gauge needle.

5.10 b) butterfly

Winged needle sets are also known as butterfly needles. They are for collecting blood from veins that are small, difficult, and close to the surface, such as veins on the back of the hand.

5.11 b) Bilirubin

Photosensitive means sensitive to light. When photosensitive analytes are exposed to light, they break down.

Bilirubin is a photosensitive analyte, as are beta-carotene, and porphyrins.

Blood samples for photosensitive analytes are collected in special tubes to prevent light from breaking down the analyte. These tubes are typically brown or amber-colored to block light from entering.

5.12 a) COPD

Pulse oximetry measures the amount of oxygen in the blood. One disease it can help monitor is chronic obstructive pulmonary disease (COPD), a lung disease that obstructs airflow and causes low oxygen levels.

5.13 c) Ear inflammation

The word otitis comes from the prefix ot- ("ear") and the suffix -itis ("inflammation").

5.14 b) A ringing sound in the ears

Tinnitus is ringing in the ears. It is a sound in the head that no one else can hear.

5.15 c) Nearsightedness

Nearsightedness (myopia) is a vision condition in which you can see objects near to you clearly, but objects farther away are blurry

5.16 a) Morning

Urine typically contains the highest concentration of hCG (human chorionic gonadotropin) in the morning. This is because urine is usually more concentrated after a night's sleep. For this reason, first-morning urine is sometimes recommended for urine pregnancy tests.

5.17 a) Arm

The PPD test involves injecting purified protein derivative (PPD) into the inner surface of the forearm. The back of the shoulder can be used if neither arm is available.

5.18 **c) PPD test**

In the PPD test, Tubersol or Aplisol are injected just under the skin. A hypersensitivity reaction indicates past or present tuberculosis.

5.19 **d) induration**

Induration is the hardening of the skin due to inflammation. Induration indicates a positive result on the PPD test.

Erythema (redness) can occur but does not by itself indicate a positive result.

5.20 **d) Tuberculosis**

The purified protein derivative (PPD) test, also known as the Mantoux test and tuberculin skin test, detects tuberculosis.

5.21 **c) Pharynx**

To obtain a specimen for a throat culture, you should swab the tonsillar area (pharynx) with a sterile cotton swab applicator.

5.22 **d) Throat**

The rapid strep test needs a swab of mucus from the back of the throat.

5.23 **c) Human chorionic gonadotropin**

Pregnancy test strips detect human chorionic gonadotropin (hCG), a hormone produced by the placenta shortly after the embryo attaches to the uterine lining. Its presence in urine or blood is an early indicator of pregnancy.

5.24 **b) invalid**

A pregnancy strip that shows no lines means the test did not work properly. Pregnancy strips have two lines: the T ("test") line and the C ("control") line. The control line should always appear because it indicates the test is functioning correctly. If the control does not appear, the test is invalid and should be thrown away.

5.25 **d) 9–10 cm**

The average distance from the nostril to the nasopharynx is 9.4 cm in women. In men, the average distance is slightly longer at 10.0 cm. This means a swab must be inserted 9–10 cm into the nasal cavity to reach the nasopharynx.

5.26 **c) Suprapubic aspiration**

Suprapubic aspiration is a procedure to take an uncontaminated urine sample to diagnose a urinary tract infection. It involves putting a needle through the skin just above the pubic bone into the bladder. It is typically used to collect urine in children who are not yet toilet trained.

5.27 **d) Urinary free cortisol test**

There are three tests for Cushing syndrome:

1. 24-hour urinary free cortisol test
2. 1-mg dexamethasone suppression test
3. Late-night salivary cortisol test

Of these, the 24-hour urinary free cortisol is usually performed first when Cushing syndrome is suspected. This test measures the amount of free (unbound) cortisol in a 24-hour urine collection. Cushing syndrome causes excessive levels of cortisol, so a high result on this test may indicate Cushing syndrome.

5.28 a) culture and susceptibility

Midstream urine samples are primarily used to look for infection.

5.29 c) HbA1c

HbA1c, also known as glycated hemoglobin, is a form of hemoglobin chemically linked to glucose. Measuring the HbA1c level gives an average of a patient's blood glucose levels over the past 2–3 months.

5.30 b) 3

When measuring the peak flow rate, three acceptable attempts must be obtained. The highest value from these attempts is then recorded as the peak flow rate.

5.31 a) L/min

The peak flow rate is measured in liters per minute and measures how quickly a patient can blow air out of their lungs. The normal range is 400–700 liters per minute.

5.32 a) As fast and hard as possible

A peak flow meter measures how much air a person can breathe out quickly. The person must take a deep breath and blow into the peak flow meter as hard and fast as possible.

5.33 d) Yellow

The yellow zone is a peak flow of 50–80% of the patient's normal peak flow. It signals caution, because the patient may be in danger of an asthma episode.

The green zone is 80–100% of the patient's normal readings and signals good health.

The red zone is <50% of the patient's normal readings and signals a medical emergency.

5.34 b) asthma

The peak flow test diagnoses asthma. The test measures how quickly a patient can blow air out of their lungs. A low score may indicate the airways are narrowed.

5.35 a) To facilitate blood sample collection

When taking a finger puncture, align the lancet at a right angle to the whorls of the fingerprint. This allows the blood to bead at the puncture site, making it easier to collect drops of blood into the container.

If you make the puncture parallel to the fingerprint whorls instead, the blood will travel down the channels between the fingerprint lines, making it difficult to collect the blood into the container.

5.36 a) Glycemia

Glycemia means the presence of glucose in the blood. Abnormal glycemia may be classified as hypoglycemia (low blood glucose) or hyperglycemia (high blood glucose).

Option b, glycogenolysis, is the breakdown of glycogen into glucose.

Option c, glycolysis, is the process by which cells break down glucose for energy.

Option d, glycosuria, is the presence of glucose in urine. Point-of-care tests measure glucose levels in the blood, not the urine.

5.37 c) Middle finger and ring finger

Finger punctures should be done on the middle finger or ring finger.

The little finger is not recommended for finger punctures because it has less tissue, increasing the risk of hitting bone during puncture.

The thumb and index finger are more sensitive than other fingers and may have calluses or scars, making them unsuitable for finger punctures.

5.38 d) Control and test

C stands for Control and T stands for Test. The control line checks if the test is working properly. The test line checks the urine for the presence of pregnancy hormones.

5.39 c) mmol/L

The SI unit for glucose tests is mmol/L.

mg/dL is the conventional unit used in the United States, not the SI unit.

5.40 a) Brownish-yellow

Jaundice is characterized by the yellowing of the skin and eyes due to high bilirubin levels in the blood. The body excretes some of the excess bilirubin in the urine, turning the urine brownish-yellow.

5.41 d) 400–700 liters per minute

Peak flow is how fast you can blow air out of your lungs. The normal adult range for peak flow is between 400 and 700 L/min.

5.42 c) Body temperature

The irrigating solution should be warmed to body temperature (37°C) for the patient's comfort.

5.43 c) Sitting up with the head tilted slightly to the side

The patient should be sitting with the head tilted in the direction of the affected ear. This allows the solution to flow out of the ear with the help of gravity.

5.44 a) A cup to collect earwax during ear irrigation

A Noots tank is a cup made of metal, plastic, or card used to catch earwax and irrigation solution during ear irrigation.

5.45 b) Dizziness

Ear irrigation may cause dizziness or vertigo. This is because the procedure may affect the balance organs in the inner ear. If the patient experiences dizziness during ear irrigation, you should stop immediately.

5.46 a) Blood glucose of 400 mg/dL

A blood glucose level of 400 mg/dL is significantly higher than the reference range of 70 to 110 mg/dL. The patient needs prompt medical attention to prevent serious health problems.

A hemoglobin of 20 g/dL is slightly high, but not an emergency.

A peak flow score of 500 L/min is a good score and indicates healthy lung function.

A positive strep test indicates a strep throat infection, typically requiring antibiotics. It is not an emergency.

5.47 a) Ears

Otoscopes (from 'oto' meaning 'ear') are devices for looking into the ears.

5.48 c) The time of the recording

On the ECG, you should include the date and time of the ECG recording, as well as the patient's name, ID number, gender, and date of birth.

5.49 a) Color blindness

The Ishihara test detects color blindness. The test uses colored plates with hidden numbers. People with normal vision can see the numbers while those with color deficiencies have difficulty seeing them.

5.50 b) 75 cm

The Ishiwara test is a color-blindness test. The test consists of 24 or 38 color plates presented one by one to the subject. The plates should be held 75 cm from the patient's face.

5.51 a) The patient can read letters from 20 feet away that most people can read from 30 feet away

20/30 vision means the patient has below-average eyesight. He has to stand 20 feet from a Snellen chart to read letters that most people can read from 30 feet away.

5.52 c) Myopia

Myopia, also known as nearsightedness, is an eye condition where close objects are clear but distant objects are blurry.

Astigmatism is blurry vision at all distances.

Hyperopia, also known as farsightedness, is the opposite of myopia: distant objects are clear but nearby objects are blurry.

Presbyopia is the gradual loss of the eyes' ability to focus on nearby objects.

5.53 d) 20 feet

A Snellen chart is placed at a standard distance of 20 feet from the patient.

5.54 c) hertz

Frequency, or pitch, is measured in hertz (Hz). A normal ear can hear a wide range of frequencies, from very low (20 Hz) to very high (20,000 Hz).

5.55 a) Frequency

The X-axis of audiograms represents sound frequency, from lowest to highest. The sounds become higher pitched as you progress from left to right.

The Y-axis measures the loudness of the sound.

5.56 c) decibels

Decibels (dB) are the unit of measurement for the loudness of sound.

5.57 d) Unilateral

Unilateral hearing loss is the medical term for hearing loss in only one ear.

5.58 a) 20–20,000 Hz

The normal range for hearing is 20–20,000 Hertz. This range encompasses a wide spectrum of sounds from low-pitched tones to high-pitched sounds.

The other options are too high for human hearing.

5.59 d) Tuning forks

Tuning forks, usually C512, are used by medical practitioners to assess a patient's hearing.

Anoscopes are used to assess problems in the anal cavity.

5.60 a) **Barrel**

The barrel of a syringe is the cylindrical part that holds the liquid. It has volume markings along its side to show how much liquid has been drawn up.

5.61 b) **Inferior**

Leads II, III, and aVF are referred to as the inferior leads because they provide a view of the inferior wall of the left ventricle.

5.62 c) **Augmented limb leads**

A standard electrocardiogram has twelve leads. Six of these leads are called limb leads because their electrodes are placed on the arms and legs of the patient. These leads are I, II, III, aVR, aVL, and aVF.

Leads I, II, and III are called bipolar limb leads because they record the differences in electrical voltage between two limbs.

Leads aVR, aVL, and aVF are called the augmented limb leads because they are created using a combination of the leads I, II and III.

5.63 b) **Lead I + Lead III = Lead II**

Einthoven's law states that the sum of the potentials of Lead I and Lead III equals that of Lead II.

5.64 b) **inferior**

Leads II, III, and aVF are called inferior leads because they observe the inferior wall of the left ventricle.

5.65 d) **Midway between V2 and V4**

Atrial fibrillation is an irregular and often fast heart rhythm.

5.66 a) **RA, LA and LL**

The electrodes RA (right arm), LA (left arm), and LL (left leg) form Einthoven's Triangle.

5.67 b) **QT**

Bazett's formula corrects the measured QT interval (the total time for ventricular depolarization and repolarization).

5.68 b) **Chest**

Electrodes V1 to V6 are all placed on the patient's chest.

5.69 a) **LA and LL**

On an ECG:

- the RA and LA electrodes form lead I
- the RA and LL electrodes form lead II
- the LA and LL electrodes form lead III

This is shown in Figure 2, which is called Einthoven's triangle.

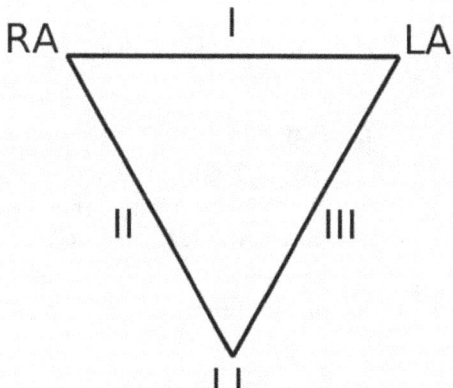

Figure 2: Einthoven's triangle.

5.70 c) Attaching the RL lead to the patient's right arm

RL means 'right leg' and should be attached to the patient's right leg, not the right arm.

5.71 a) Atrial flutter

The lead positions shown in the diagram are called the Lewis lead method. This method is useful in diagnosing atrial flutter because it provides a focused view of the atria.

5.72 a) LA and RA

Lead I produces a tracing representing the voltage difference between the left arm (LA) and the right arm (RA).

This is shown in the Einthoven triangle in Figure 3.

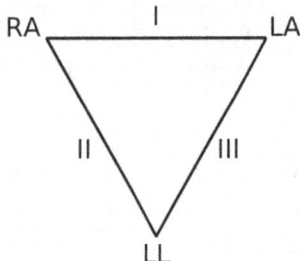

Figure 3: The Einthoven triangle.

5.73 d) Tachycardia

Tachycardia is a heart rate over 100 beats per minute. For patients with tachycardia, you may need to increase the ECG paper speed from 25 mm/sec to 50 mm/sec to make the output easier to read.

5.74 d) Place the LL electrode above the patient's left knee instead

Since you cannot place the LL electrode on the patient's lower left leg, you should place the electrode on the upper left leg instead, or on the lower torso anywhere caudal to the heart. Since the EKG measures electrical vectors, it does not matter whether the arm or leg electrode is on the arm or leg; they just have to be relatively close to the line drawn between the heart and the limb.

5.75 b) b

The LA lead is placed on the patient's left arm.

5.76 c) At the fourth intercostal space, right sternal border

The V1 lead is placed at the fourth intercostal space at the right sternal border.

5.77 b) To attach alligator clips

ECG electrodes have tabs to facilitate the attachment of alligator clips, which are part of the leads that connect the electrodes to the ECG machine.

5.78 d) augmented

AVL stands for 'augmented voltage left'. Left in this case means the left arm.

5.79 d) Stop the test

If the patient starts showing signs of cardiac ischemia (such as severe shortness of breath or chest pain), the test must be stopped immediately to prevent further complications.

5.80 **a) Alcohol wipes are used to clean the skin**

Alcohol wipes are used to remove dirt particles that may cause any signal interference with the electrodes. Soap and water may also be used.

Option b is incorrect because shaving the patient's entire chest is not necessary. Shaving only the areas where the electrodes will be attached is necessary, and even then, only if the patient has a hairy chest.

Option c is incorrect because patients are not required to fast before an ECG.

Option d is incorrect because the patient should be lying down, not seated.

5.81 **b) At the fourth intercostal space to the left of the sternum**

The V2 lead is placed at the fourth intercostal space to the left of the sternum (breastbone).

5.82 **a) 25 mm/second**

25 mm/second is the normal paper speed for an ECG, though 50 mm/second may be used if the ECG cycles are too close together.

5.83 **c) Obtain the patient's consent**

When performing an ECG, the first step is to explain the procedure to the patient and obtain their consent. Touching a patient without their consent can give rise to legal charges, and even allegations of battery or assault.

5.84 **d) RL**

RL stands for 'right leg'.

5.85 **b) N**

The right leg electrode is also known as the N electrode (for 'neutral').

F (for 'foot') is another name for the left leg electrode.

5.86 **b) Green**

The neutral electrode is green and marked with the letters RL (right leg).

5.87 **a) To facilitate conductivity between the skin and the electrode**

The human skin has a high resistance to electrical signals, which can interfere with the accuracy of the ECG recording. Applying a conductive substance (like paste or jelly) to the skin reduces this resistance, allowing the heart's electrical signals to be transmitted more effectively to the ECG electrodes.

5.88 **d) White**

In the American Heart Association ECG lead color coding system:

- the RA electrode is white
- the LA electrode is black
- the RL electrode is green
- the LL electrode is red

5.89 **c) Lateral**

Leads I, aVL, V5, and V6 are the lateral leads as they provide a view of the lateral wall of the left ventricle.

5.90 **b) Lead II**

The QT interval is best measured in lead II.

5.91 **d) aVR**

aVR is the augmented unipolar right arm lead. It is called "augmented" because its signal is amplified, and "unipolar" because it records activity from one electrode on the right arm.

5.92 b) bipolar

The six limb leads are I, II, III, aVR, aVL, and aVF. Three are unipolar (aVR, aVL, and aVF) and three are bipolar (I, II, and III).

5.93 b) II

Lead II, which usually gives a good view of the P wave, is most commonly used to record the rhythm strip.

5.94 d) RA and LL

Lead I is the difference between the right arm (RA) and left arm (LA) electrodes.

Lead II is the difference between the right arm (RA) and left leg (LL) electrodes.

Lead III is the difference between the left leg (LL) and left arm (LA) electrodes.

This is shown the Einthoven triangle in Figure 4.

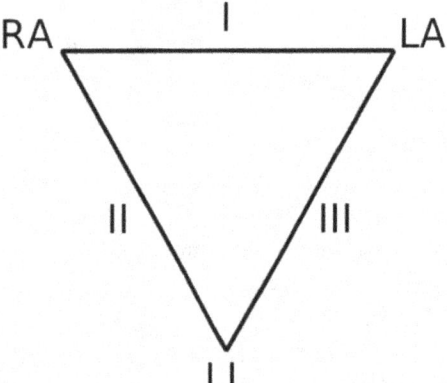

Figure 4: The Einthoven triangle.

5.95 c) chest

Leads V1 to V6 are called the chest leads because their electrodes are placed on the chest. Leads I, II, III, aVR, aVL, and aVF are called the limb leads because they are created from electrodes placed on the arms and legs.

5.96 d) The midaxillary line at the same level as V4 and V5

V6 is placed at the midaxillary line at the same horizontal level as V4 and V5.

5.97 a) 10 mm

A normal standardization mark on an ECG tracing is typically 10 mm (1 cm) in height. The standardization mark is a calibration point that is used to ensure that the ECG machine is recording the electrical activity of the heart accurately. It is a vertical line that appears on the ECG paper and serves as a reference point for measuring the amplitude (height) of the ECG waves and complexes.

5.98 b) Baseline wander

Baseline wander in an ECG is the slow, wandering movements of the baseline. Typically, the entire signal moves up and down as a gradual, undulating wave. The cause is usually the patient's breathing.

5.99 d) Muscle tremor

Muscle tremor artifacts look like erratic spikes on the ECG tracing. They happen when the patient is shivering or propping themselves up on their arms.

5.100 a) AC interference

AC interference looks like a thick, fuzzy line on the ECG tracing. It results from nearby electrical devices such as laptops, tablets, and phones.

Content Area 6

Administering Medications/Vaccines

There are 52 questions in this content area.

6.1 Levothyroxine is the treatment for which disorder?
   a) Hypertension
   b) Hyperthyroidism
   c) Hypotension
   d) Hypothyroidism

6.2 Vaccination is what type of immunity?
   a) Artificial active
   b) Artificial passive
   c) Natural active
   d) Natural passive

6.3 At what temperature are vaccines stored?
   a) −18°C and below
   b) 2–8°C
   c) Room temperature
   d) 36–37.5°C

6.4 Which vaccine is recommended during pregnancy?
   a) HPV
   b) Tdap
   c) Typhoid fever
   d) Varicella

Answers on page 84

6.5 The MMR vaccine protects against which three diseases?
   a) Malaria, measles, and roseola
   b) Malaria, meningitis, and rabies
   c) Mumps, measles, and rubella
   d) Mumps, meningitis, and rickets

6.6 Which needle gauge is used to administer intramuscular vaccines to children?
   a) 22–25
   b) 23–26
   c) 24–27
   d) 25–28

6.7 Some vaccines come as "lyophilized" powders. What does lyophilized mean?
   a) Freeze-dried
   b) Irradiated with non-ionizing radiation
   c) Sprayed with preservatives
   d) Sterilized

6.8 Which disease has a vaccine that can be administered by the intranasal route?
   a) COVID-19
   b) Influenza
   c) Rotavirus
   d) Tuberculosis

6.9 Immunocompromised patients can safely receive which of these vaccines?
   a) MMR
   b) Rotavirus
   c) Tdap
   d) Zostavax

6.10 At what age is the first dose of varicella vaccine given?
   a) 12–15 months
   b) 2–3 years
   c) 4–6 years
   d) 7–10 years

Answers on page 84

6.11 Which of these vaccines requires reconstitution before administration?
   a) Hepatitis B
   b) Influenza
   c) Tetanus
   d) Varicella

6.12 Vaccines injected into the same limb must be spaced at least _____ apart.
   a) 0.5 inches
   b) 1 inch
   c) 1.5 inches
   d) 2 inches

6.13 What needle size is used to administer intramuscular vaccines to adults?
   a) 22–25 gauge, 1–1.5 inches
   b) 16–18 gauge, 1/2 inch
   c) 25–27 gauge, 3/8 inch
   d) 30–32 gauge, 1 inch

6.14 Which of these vaccines is administered orally?
   a) Hepatitis B
   b) Rotavirus
   c) Rubella
   d) Tetanus

6.15 Which type of vaccine uses killed bacteria?
   a) Inactivated
   b) Live-attenuated
   c) Toxoid
   d) Viral-vector

6.16 What do Vaccine Information Statements explain?
   a) How patients can self-administer vaccines at home
   b) Insurance coverage details for vaccines
   c) The benefits and risks of a vaccine
   d) The requirements for handling and storing a vaccine

Answers on page 85

6.17 Which of these is a contraindication for the MMR vaccination?
- a) Current use of antibiotics
- b) Hayfever
- c) Low-grade fever
- d) Pregnancy

6.18 Which of these is a common side effect of vaccines?
- a) Fever
- b) Hunger
- c) Thirst
- d) Wheezing

6.19 By what route are suppositories administered?
- a) Inhalation
- b) Parenteral
- c) Rectal
- d) Topical

6.20 Antiemetic medications help to treat which health problem?
- a) Cancer
- b) Constipation
- c) Migraine
- d) Nausea

6.21 What do vasodilators do?
- a) Decrease glucose levels
- b) Increase the activity of neurotransmitters in the brain
- c) Inhibit the metabolism of glucose
- d) Widen blood vessels

6.22 What is the term for a drug that contains the same chemical substance as a brand-name drug?
- a) Controlled
- b) Generic
- c) Over-the-counter
- d) Prescription

Answers on page 85

6.23 Haloperidol is a medication used to treat which health problem?
   a) Hypertension
   b) Insomnia
   c) Rheumatoid arthritis
   d) Schizophrenia

6.24 Which of these medications is a mood stabilizer for treating bipolar disorder?
   a) Dihydrocodeine
   b) Doxazosin
   c) Epinephrine
   d) Lithium

6.25 Which of these medications is an anabolic steroid?
   a) Albuterol
   b) Anadrol
   c) Librium
   d) Vicodin

6.26 Nitroglycerin is a:
   a) anti-hypertensive
   b) cardiotonic
   c) diuretic
   d) vasodilator

6.27 Which of these medications lowers the level of LDL cholesterol in the blood?
   a) Beta-blockers
   b) Corticosteroids
   c) Diuretics
   d) Statins

6.28 Which cardiac glycoside is used to treat congenital heart failure and arrhythmias by increasing cardiac output?
   a) Digoxin
   b) Furosemide
   c) Minoxidil
   d) Spironolactone

Answers on page 86

6.29 How are aerosols administered?
   a) As a topical gel
   b) By inhalation
   c) By rectal administration
   d) Parenterally

6.30 Drugs that block release of a substance that causes allergic reactions are called:
   a) anticoagulants
   b) anticonvulsants
   c) antidiabetics
   d) antihistamines

6.31 Which type of drug increases urine output?
   a) Barbiturate
   b) Corticosteroid
   c) Diuretic
   d) Immunosuppressant

6.32 Which drugs relieve allergy symptoms?
   a) Anticoagulants
   b) Anticonvulsants
   c) Antidiabetics
   d) Antihistamines

6.33 Drugs that produce loss of sensation are called:
   a) analgesics
   b) anesthetics
   c) anticonvulsants
   d) tranquilizers

6.34 Which of these medication combinations could cause hyperkalemia (high blood potassium)?
   a) Diazepam and oxycodone
   b) Digoxin and verapamil
   c) Fluoxetine and phenelzine
   d) Lisinopril and spironolactone

Answers on page 87

6.35 Penicillin, amoxicillin, and ciprofloxacin are examples of which type of drug?
   a) Antibiotics
   b) Anticoagulants
   c) Antihistamines
   d) Antivirals

6.36 Acetaminophen is used to treat:
   a) allergies and itching
   b) fever and pain
   c) heartburn and acid reflux
   d) infection and inflammation

6.37 What does the pharmaceutical abbreviation QDS mean?
   a) Every day
   b) Every four hours
   c) Every hour
   d) Four times a day

6.38 What is the pharmacy abbreviation for the right ear?
   a) AD
   b) AS
   c) ASA
   d) AU

6.39 What does the pharmaceutical abbreviation "pc" mean?
   a) After meals
   b) At bedtime
   c) Before meals
   d) In the morning

6.40 What angle is used for a subcutaneous injection on thin patients?
   a) 15°
   b) 30°
   c) 45°
   d) 90°

Answers on page 87

6.41 The five rights of medication administration are right person, right medicine, right route, right dose, and:
   a) right physician
   b) right result
   c) right time
   d) right to refuse

6.42 The Z-track method is used for which type of injection?
   a) Intramuscular
   b) Intrathecal
   c) Intravenous
   d) Subcutaneous

6.43 What is the most common site for intramuscular injection in adults?
   a) Abdomen
   b) Anterolateral thigh
   c) Deltoid
   d) Triceps

6.44 How should you dispose of a needle after administering an injection?
   a) Leave the needle uncapped and place it in a biohazard bag
   b) Leave the needle uncapped and place it in a sharps disposal container
   c) Recap the needle and place it in a biohazard bag
   d) Recap the needle and place it in a sharps disposal container

6.45 If a patient needs to take 20 mg of a medication per day for 1 week, and the medication comes in 10 mg tablets, how many tablets should the patient take per day?
   a) 1
   b) 2
   c) 3
   d) 4

Answers on page 88

6.46 A patient must take an extended-release medication but has difficulty swallowing the tablet because of its size. What should you do?
   a) Contact the provider to discuss an alternate form of the medication
   b) Crush the tablet
   c) Cut the tablet in half
   d) Dissolve the tablet in water

6.47 A doctor orders a medication of 1 g/kg of body weight. If the patient weighs 181 lb, how many grams of the medication should be given?
   a) 81 g
   b) 91g
   c) 108 g
   d) 181 g

6.48 What angle is used for subcutaneous injections on obese patients?
   a) 15°
   b) 30°
   c) 45°
   d) 90°

6.49 How is NPH insulin administered?
   a) Intramuscularly
   b) Intravenously
   c) Orally
   d) Subcutaneously

6.50 In California, which of these can a medical assistant legally inject into a patient?
   a) Anesthetics
   b) Chemotherapy medication
   c) Collagen
   d) Narcotics

Answers on page 88

6.51 Which of these needles is appropriate for an intramuscular injection?
   a) 16 G, 2.5 inch
   b) 20 G, 2 inch
   c) 24 G, 1.5 inch
   d) 28 G, 1 inch

6.52 A patient requires a dose of 12.5 mg but the medication is only available in 100 mg/2 mL ampules. How many mL should the patient take?
   a) 0.125
   b) 0.25
   c) 0.5
   d) 1

Answers on page 89

ANSWERS

6.1 d) Hypothyroidism

Levothyroxine is a medication used to treat an underactive thyroid gland (hypothyroidism).

6.2 a) Artificial active

Vaccines provide artificial active immunity. The immunity is active because the person's body makes its own antibodies to the disease. This is in contrast to passive immunization, where antibodies are made by another human being or animal.

Furthermore, the immunity is artificial because the vaccine is given intentionally, before the person has natural exposure to the disease. The alternative to artificial immunization is natural immunization, where a person is infected by a pathogen.

6.3 b) 2–8°C

Most vaccines are refrigerated at 2–8°C to maintain their effectiveness.

6.4 b) Tdap

The two vaccines recommended during pregnancy are the inactivated flu vaccine and the Tdap vaccine. The Tdap vaccine protects against tetanus, diphtheria, and pertussis.

6.5 c) Mumps, measles, and rubella

The MMR vaccine is a combination vaccine protecting against mumps, measles, and rubella, which are contagious viral diseases.

6.6 a) 22–25

A needle gauge of 22 to 25 is recommended for intramuscular injection. This applies to people of all ages, from neonates to adults.

6.7 a) Freeze-dried

Lyophilized means "freeze-dried". Freeze-drying is a process that removes water by turning it from ice to vapor. The process helps preserve vaccines.

6.8 b) Influenza

The only vaccine available in an intranasal spray format is FluMist, a vaccine against influenza.

6.9 c) Tdap

Immunocompromised patients can safely receive inactivated vaccines. The tetanus, diphtheria, and pertussis (Tdap) vaccine is an inactivated vaccine.

Live vaccines, such as MMR (Measles, Mumps, Rubella) and Zostavax, are not recommended for immunocompromised patients due to the risk of causing disease.

6.10 a) 12–15 months

The first dose of varicella vaccine is given at 12–15 months and the second dose is given at 4–6 years.

6.11 d) Varicella

Varicella (chickenpox) vaccine requires reconstitution before administration. This vaccine comes as a powder that needs to be mixed with a liquid before injection.

Vaccines against influenza, hepatitis B, and tetanus come as pre-filled syringes or vials containing the liquid vaccine ready for injection.

6.12 b) 1 inch

Two vaccines administered in a single limb must be spaced at least an inch apart, to reduce the potential for swelling and pain.

6.13 a) 22–25 gauge, 1–1.5 inches

For most adults, a 22–25 gauge 1–1.5 inch needle is used for intramuscular administration.

6.14 b) Rotavirus

Rotavirus vaccines are only available for oral administration. They are not injected.

6.15 a) Inactivated

Inactivated vaccines contain killed bacteria or inactivated viruses. This allows the body to develop immunity without getting the actual disease.

Live-attenuated vaccines use weakened (attenuated) versions of live viruses or bacteria.

Toxoid vaccines contain the toxins produced by bacteria, not the bacteria themselves.

Viral vector vaccines use a virus to provide the body with instructions to produce antigens. The body's cells then create these antigens, triggering an immune response.

6.16 c) The benefits and risks of a vaccine

Vaccine Information Statements inform patients about the benefits and risks of a vaccine they are about to receive.

6.17 d) Pregnancy

The MMR is a live-attenuated vaccine. It is not recommended during pregnancy because of the potential risk the vaccine could infect the unborn baby.

6.18 a) Fever

Out of the choices, fever is a common side effect of vaccines. Vaccinations activate the immune system, causing mild fever. Fever will usually resolve within a day or two.

6.19 c) Rectal

Suppositories are administered rectally. They melt in the rectum and release their medicine. Once melted, the medication is absorbed into the bloodstream.

Inhalation refers to the administration of medication by the lungs.

Parenteral means administered by a route other than the mouth and alimentary canal, such as by injection.

Topical refers to the application of medication to the skin.

6.20 d) Nausea

Antiemetics are drugs that prevent or reduce nausea and vomiting.

6.21 d) Widen blood vessels

Vasodilators are medications that dilate (widen) blood vessels.

6.22 b) Generic

Generic drugs are drugs with the same active ingredients as brand-name drugs, but they usually cost less than brand-name drugs.

6.23 d) Schizophrenia

Haloperidol is an antipsychotic used to treat schizophrenia.

6.24 d) Lithium

Lithium is used to treat episodes of mania in people with bipolar disorder.

Dihydrocodeine is an opioid used to treat pain.

Doxazosin is used to treat high blood pressure and symptoms of an enlarged prostate.

Epinephrine, more commonly known as adrenaline, is used to treat severe allergic reactions (anaphylaxis) and asthma attacks.

6.25 b) Anadrol

Anabolic steroids are synthetic (man-made) versions of testosterone. Oxymetholone, sold under the brand name Anadrol (among others), is an example of an anabolic steroid.

Albuterol is a bronchodilator used to treat asthma and other respiratory conditions.

Librium is a benzodiazepine used for anxiety and insomnia.

Vicodin is an opioid pain medication.

6.26 d) vasodilator

Nitroglycerin is a vasodilatory drug used primarily to provide relief from anginal chest pain. Vasodilators are a group of medicines that dilate (open) blood vessels, which allows blood to flow more easily.

6.27 d) Statins

Statins are medicines that lower the level of low-density lipoprotein (LDL) cholesterol in the blood.

Option a, beta-blockers, slow down the heart by blocking the action of hormones like adrenaline.

Option b, corticosteroids, are an anti-inflammatory medicine.

Option c, diuretics, increase urine output.

6.28 a) Digoxin

Digoxin is a cardiac glycoside used to treat heart failure and certain arrhythmias. It works by increasing the force of heart muscle contractions, thereby improving cardiac output.

6.29 b) By inhalation

Aerosols are administered by inhalation, meaning they are breath in through the nose or mouth.

6.30 d) antihistamines

Antihistamines are medications that block the release of histamine, a substance involved in allergic reactions. Histamine causes symptoms like sneezing, runny nose, itchy eyes, and hives. By blocking the effects of histamine, antihistamines help alleviate these symptoms.

6.31 c) Diuretic

Diuretics make the kidneys produce more urine. They are often used to treat high blood pressure.

Barbiturates are depressants that make you feel relaxed and drowsy.

Corticosteroids are anti-inflammatories. They are used to treat inflammation and autoimmune disorders.

Immunosuppressants suppress the immune system. They are used in organ transplant recipients and people with autoimmune diseases.

6.32 d) Antihistamines

Antihistamines are the most common drugs that treat allergies. They block histamine, the chemical that causes allergy symptoms.

6.33 b) anesthetics

Drugs that produce a loss of sensation are called anesthetics. They are used to prevent pain during surgeries.

6.34 d) Lisinopril and spironolactone

Lisinopril and spironolactone are medications used to treat high blood pressure and certain heart conditions. They both have the side effect of increasing potassium levels. When taken together, the side effect is additive, increasing the risk of high potassium levels.

The other medication combinations cause other problems:

Both diazepam and oxycodone depress the central nervous system. Taking both together can cause severe respiratory depression, leading to death.

Verapamil increases digoxin concentration in the blood. Taking verapamil and digoxin together could therefore cause digoxin toxicity.

Fluoxetine and phenelzine both increase serotonin levels. Taking both drugs together can cause a potentially life-threatening condition called serotonin syndrome.

6.35 a) Antibiotics

Penicillin, amoxicillin, and ciprofloxacin are antibiotics. Antibiotics treat bacterial infections by killing or inhibiting the growth of bacteria.

6.36 b) fever and pain

Acetaminophen (commonly known as paracetamol) is used to treat fever and pain.

6.37 d) Four times a day

QDS stands for *quater die sumendus* which is Latin for "four times a day." When used on a prescription, QDS means the prescribed medication should be taken four times a day.

The abbreviation for every day is QD (*quaque die,* meaning "every hour").

The abbreviation for every four hours is Q4H (*quaque 4 hora,* meaning "every four hours").

The abbreviation for every hour is QH (*quaque hora,* meaning "every hour").

6.38 a) AD

AD is derived from Latin "auris dextra" and means "right ear".

AS means left ear.

ASA means aspirin.

AU means both ears.

6.39 a) After meals

pc (post cibum) means "after meals".

6.40 c) 45°

Subcutaneous injections are given into the fat under the skin. For normal-sized or obese patients, an angle of 90 degrees is used. For thin patients, however, an angle of 45 degrees is used instead, to ensure the needle does not go through the fat.

6.41 c) right time

The five rights of medication administration help to prevent errors when administering drugs to patients. The five rights are:

1. Right patient (does the order match the patient?)
2. Right medicine (is the medication correct?)
3. Right route (are you using the correct route of administration?)
4. Right dose (do you have the correct dose?)
5. Right time (are you giving the drug at the correct time?)

6.42 a) Intramuscular

The Z-track injection technique is used for intramuscular injections. The technique helps prevent medications from leaking into the subcutaneous tissue layer.

6.43 c) Deltoid

The deltoid muscle is the preferred injection site for adults and children aged 3–18. The deltoid muscles are in the shoulders.

The anterolateral thigh is preferred for newborns and infants since their deltoids are not large enough.

6.44 b) Leave the needle uncapped and place it in a sharps disposal container

Used needles should be placed in a sharps disposal container. Don't recap the needle as you could accidentally puncture yourself.

6.45 b) 2

$$\frac{20 \text{ mg}}{10 \text{ mg per tablet}} = 2 \text{ tablets}$$

6.46 a) Contact the provider to discuss an alternate form of the medication

Extended-release tablets should never be crushed, cut or dissolved. Doing so will release the drug into the body too early.

6.47 a) 81 g

To convert pounds to kilograms, divide the number of pounds by 2.205:

$$\frac{181}{2.205} = 82 \text{ kilograms}$$

Since the ratio of medication to weight is 1 g/kg, the amount of the medication needed is 82 g.

6.48 d) 90°

For obese and normal-sized patients, a 90-degree angle is used for subcutaneous injections. This angle helps ensure the medication reaches the subcutaneous tissue layer beneath the skin.

Thinner patients require an angle of 45 degrees to ensure the needle does not go through the fat.

6.49 d) Subcutaneously

NPH (neutral protamine Hagedorn) insulin is administered by subcutaneous injection only.

6.50 d) Narcotics

In California, medical assistants can administer injections of scheduled drugs (including narcotics), as long as:

1. a licensed physician verifies the dosage and supervises the procedure, and
2. the injection is administered intramuscularly, subcutaneously, or intradermally (not intravenously)

6.51 c) 24 G, 1.5 inch

Intramuscular injections require 22-25 gauge needles 1-1.5 inches long (up to 3 inches for large adults).

6.52 b) 0.25

First, calculate the amount of medication per milliliter:

$$\frac{100 \text{ mg}}{2 \text{ mL}} = 50 \text{ mg/mL}$$

Next, calculate how many mL contain 12.5 mg:

$$\frac{12.5 \text{ mg}}{50 \text{ mg/mL}} = 0.25 \text{ mL}$$

Content Area 7

Discharging Patients

There are 15 questions in this content area.

7.1 After a blood draw, patients should avoid:
   a) driving
   b) eating a large meal
   c) heavy lifting
   d) lying down

7.2 Sutures and staples should be removed within:
   a) 1–2 hours
   b) 7–10 hours
   c) 1–2 days
   d) 7–10 days

7.3 Which of these terms would patients most easily understand?
   a) Dilation
   b) Erythema
   c) Purpura
   d) Redness

Answers on page 94

7.4 Patients with heart disease should lower their intake of:
a) calcium
b) iron
c) potassium
d) sodium

7.5 Which of these is a care instruction for a mother of a baby with mild jaundice?
a) Administer oral vitamin K drops 3 times per day
b) Breastfeed your baby often
c) Do not let your baby sleep for more than 2 hours at a time
d) Keep your baby in a dimly lit area

7.6 A patient receives general anesthetic for an operation. After the operation, a medical assistant needs to discharge the patient home. What instruction should the medical assistant give to the patient?
a) Do not drive for 24 hours
b) Drink 2 liters of sugary drinks over the next 12 hours to replenish electrolytes
c) Take a hot bath
d) Take a laxative every other day to avoid constipation

7.7 A patient has had cryosurgery to remove a skin lesion. Which of these is the correct aftercare instruction?
a) Apply glycolic acid cream every 6–8 hours
b) Open the blister should one appear
c) Scrub the site softly with a brush once a day
d) Use a cool compress to relieve discomfort

7.8 Which of the following is a correct aftercare instruction for a urinary tract infection?
a) Drink plenty of caffeine
b) Take antibiotics as directed
c) Urinate as little as possible
d) Wipe from back to front after using the toilet

Answers on page 94

7.9 Which of these would be found in an after visit summary?
  a) Billing information
  b) Family history
  c) Follow-up care instructions
  d) Insurance details

7.10 When should patients receive an after visit summary?
  a) After every visit
  b) Every 3 months
  c) Every 6 months
  d) Every 12 months

7.11 A medical assistant is giving discharge instructions to a patient hospitalized with pneumonia. Which of these replies indicates the patient has misunderstood the instructions?
  a) "I can start eating a normal diet right away"
  b) "I can stop taking antibiotics once my symptoms have gone"
  c) "I should go home and get rest"
  d) "I should keep using the incentive spirometer to keep my airways open"

7.12 What is the purpose of an after visit summary?
  a) To notify the patient's family about the visit
  b) To remind the patient what they discussed with their doctor
  c) To schedule future appointments
  d) To update the patient's insurance information

7.13 Which medication would an immunocompromised patient receive after wound debridement?
  a) Antibiotic
  b) Bronchodilator
  c) Corticosteroid
  d) Sedative

Answers on page 95

7.14 What is the main purpose of a discharge summary report?
   a) To communicate a patient's care plan to the post-hospital care team
   b) To document legal issues that arose during the hospitalization
   c) To justify the hospitalisation costs to the insurance company
   d) To summarize the costs incurred during the patient's hospitalization

7.15 Which of these is included in a discharge summary report?
   a) Detailed daily progress notes
   b) Diagnostic images
   c) Patient's insurance details
   d) Reason for admission

Answers on page 95

ANSWERS

7.1 c) heavy lifting

Strenuous activity like heavy lifting can increase pressure at the blood draw site and cause more bleeding.

7.2 d) 7–10 days

Sutures and staples are typically removed after 7 to 10 days. This is enough time for the wound to heal in most cases.

7.3 d) Redness

Patients may not understand medical terms, so it is best to use everyday words where possible.

7.4 d) sodium

Sodium (salt) can cause the body to retain fluid, which increases blood pressure and makes the heart work harder, which can be dangerous for patients with heart disease.

Potassium lowers the risk of cardiovascular disease.

7.5 b) Breastfeed your baby often

An excess of bilirubin causes jaundice. The fluids from breastfeeding help the baby's liver to remove the extra bilirubin.

7.6 a) Do not drive for 24 hours

Patients should refrain from driving for 24 to 48 hours after general anesthesia. This is because general anesthesia impairs the senses and increases the risk of a car accident.

7.7 d) Use a cool compress to relieve discomfort

The wound can hurt after cryosurgery. To reduce pain and inflammation, the patient should use a cool compress or ice pack for 2–3 minutes several times an hour.

The patient should avoid creams containing glycolic acid, vitamin C, or retinol creams for 7–10 days after cryosurgery.

7.8 b) Take antibiotics as directed

Patients with a urinary tract infection should take antibiotics as directed to kill the infection.

Drinking caffeine with a urinary tract infection is not recommended. Caffeine can irritate the bladder and worsen symptoms.

Urinating as little as possible is incorrect. Patients with a urinary tract infection should urinate frequently. The longer they hold urine, the higher the risk for bacteria to build up in their system.

Wiping from back to front after using the toilet is not advised. Doing this can spread feces into the vagina. It is always recommended to wipe from front to back instead.

7.9 c) Follow-up care instructions

After visit summaries typically contain:

- reason for the visit
- vital signs for the visit
- diagnoses
- tests ordered
- key findings from the test results

- medications and treatments ordered
- follow-up care instructions
- recommendations

7.10 a) After every visit

Patients should receive an after-visit summary after every medical appointment. This document provides an overview of the visit and may include the diagnosis, treatment plan, medications, and follow-up appointments.

7.11 b) "I can stop taking antibiotics once my symptoms have gone"

The patient must complete the entire course of antibiotics, even if symptoms improve earlier. Stopping antibiotics prematurely can mean incomplete eradication of the infection.

7.12 b) To remind the patient what they discussed with their doctor

An after visit summary is a document given to patients after a medical appointment. It is intended to help patients better understand and remember what they have discussed with their doctor.

7.13 a) Antibiotic

An immunocompromised patient would likely receive an antibiotic after wound debridement to prevent infection.

7.14 a) To communicate a patient's care plan to the post-hospital care team

The discharge summary is a summary of what happened to the patient in the hospital. Its purpose is to document information needed by the patient's primary care physician for continuity of care.

7.15 d) Reason for admission

Discharge summary reports provide a brief overview of a patient's hospitalization. These reports include information such as:

- reason for admission
- examination findings
- response to treatment
- condition of the patient on discharge
- discharge diagnosis
- recommendations for follow-up

"Detailed daily progress notes" is incorrect because the summary should include an overview of the patient's progress, not detailed daily notes.

"Diagnostic images" is incorrect because while the discharge summary might describe significant imaging findings, it does not include the actual images.

"Patient's insurance details" is incorrect because discharge summaries do not include financial and insurance information.

Content Area 8

Responding to Codes/Emergencies

There are 27 questions in this content area.

8.1 What is the medical term for a heart attack?
   a) Angina
   b) Angina pectoris
   c) Cardiomyopathy
   d) Myocardial infarction

8.2 Insulin overdose causes which of these diabetic emergencies?
   a) Diabetic ketoacidosis
   b) Diabetic neuropathy
   c) Diabetic retinopathy
   d) Diabetic shock

8.3 What is the first step in caring for a wound with heavy bleeding?
   a) Add bulky dressings to reinforce blood-soaked bandages
   b) Apply direct pressure with a sterile dressing
   c) Apply pressure at a pressure point
   d) Ask the casualty to recite the alphabet

Answers on page 102

8.4 A patient appears to be intoxicated. Her speech is incoherent. Her breathing is rapid. Her pulse is 120. Around her wrist is a diabetic medical bracelet. Which of these actions would be the most appropriate?
   a) Give the patient a glass of water
   b) Give the patient a sugary drink
   c) Give the patient time to recover on her own
   d) Inject the patient with insulin

8.5 The recovery position is used for patients who are:
   a) breathing abnormally
   b) unconscious and not breathing
   c) unconscious but breathing normally
   d) undergoing cardiac arrest

8.6 Activated charcoal is used to treat:
   a) asthma
   b) convulsions
   c) hypotension
   d) poisoning

8.7 In stroke recognition, what does the acronym FAST stand for?
   a) Face, arm, speech and time
   b) Fever, anxiety, stress, and taste
   c) First airway, second temperature
   d) Flexibility, asthma, and sudden tightness

8.8 In CPR, how many chest compressions should be given per second?
   a) 1
   b) 2
   c) 3
   d) 4

Answers on page 103

8.9 The rule of nines indicates the:
   a) amount of IV fluid necessary
   b) amount of infection present
   c) depth of a burn
   d) percentage of body area affected by a burn

8.10 What should you do if someone is having a seizure?
   a) Give mouth-to-mouth breaths
   b) Hold them down
   c) Put something soft under their head
   d) Put something wooden in their mouth

8.11 First aid for a snake bite to the arm includes:
   a) Applying a tourniquet
   b) Applying ice to the injury
   c) Immobilizing the arm
   d) Sucking the venom out of the wound

8.12 When should you NEVER administer care to a casualty?
   a) When the person has stopped breathing
   b) When the person is having a seizure
   c) When the person is unconscious
   d) When the person refuses care

8.13 A patient presents with hives, difficulty breathing, and sneezing. What is the most likely cause?
   a) Anaphylactic shock
   b) Heart attack
   c) Insulin overdose
   d) Stroke

8.14 How many inches deep are chest compressions for CPR?
   a) 1
   b) 2
   c) 3
   d) 4

Answers on page 104

8.15 Which of the following is the correct sequence of events in the chain of survival?
   a) Call 911 → defibrillation → start CPR
   b) Call 911 → start CPR → defibrillation
   c) Defibrillation → call 911 → start CPR
   d) Start CPR → call 911 → defibrillation

8.16 Where on the patient should you place your hands for CPR?
   a) The center of the chest
   b) The diaphragm
   c) The pelvis
   d) The stomach

8.17 What does ABC stand for in first aid?
   a) Active body control
   b) Airway, breathing, and circulation
   c) Always be careful
   d) Attention, beware, check

8.18 A patient has frostbite in his fingers. What measure can you take before transporting the patient to emergency care?
   a) Apply a heating pad
   b) Immerse his hands in hot water
   c) Loosely wrap his fingers in bandages
   d) Rub his hands vigorously

8.19 How do you care for someone with a possible neck injury?
   a) Ask the person to try to move their head
   b) Keep the person's head still and do not try to move it
   c) Move the person into a comfortable position
   d) Move the person's head so that it rests above their heart

Answers on page 105

8.20 The chain of survival is a four-step process that can help save the lives of victims of:
   a) cardiac arrest
   b) diabetic coma
   c) massive blood loss
   d) stroke

8.21 When administering CPR, give:
   a) 40 compressions followed by 1 breath
   b) 30 compressions followed by 2 breaths
   c) 20 compressions followed by 5 breaths
   d) 10 compressions followed by 10 breaths

8.22 A colleague has cut his lower arm and is bleeding. Which of the following is NOT an appropriate response?
   a) Apply firm pressure to the wound using sterile gauze
   b) Clean and dress the wound once the bleeding has stopped
   c) Place a tourniquet over the elbow joint
   d) Wear gloves

8.23 The Heimlich maneuver is used for:
   a) choking
   b) heart attack
   c) poisoning
   d) syncope

8.24 Which four medications are stored on crash carts for breathing emergencies?
   a) Alprazolam, carisoprodol, clonazepam, and clorazepate
   b) Amphetamine, methamphetamine, methylphenidate, and amobarbital
   c) Hydromorphone, methadone, meperidine, and oxycodone
   d) Terbutaline, epinephrine, aminophylline, and albuterol

Answers on page 105

8.25 Which of these patients should be attended to first?
   a) A boy with a minor bite from a dog that was vaccinated against rabies
   b) A man who had knee replacement surgery three days ago and now has swelling and pain in his leg
   c) A woman complaining of nausea twelve hours after a hysterectomy
   d) A woman with a temperature of 99.9°F

8.26 Which medication is used in an emergency to stop convulsions and seizures?
   a) Diazepam
   b) Epinephrine
   c) Nitroprusside
   d) Terbutaline

8.27 Which hospital emergency code is used for adults going into cardiac arrest?
   a) Blue
   b) Gray
   c) Red
   d) Yellow

Answers on page 106

ANSWERS

8.1 d) Myocardial infarction

Myocardial infarction is the medical term for a heart attack. It occurs when a coronary artery becomes blocked, reducing blood flow to the heart muscle.

Option a, angina (also known as angina pectoris), is chest pain due to part of the heart not getting enough blood and oxygen.

Option c, cardiomyopathy, is a general term for diseases of the heart muscle, in which the heart loses its ability to pump blood effectively.

8.2 d) Diabetic shock

Diabetic shock, also known as insulin shock or hypoglycemic shock, occurs when a diabetic takes too much insulin. This causes their blood glucose levels to drop too low.

Diabetic ketoacidosis is when a lack of insulin causes harmful substances called ketones to build up in the blood. Insulin overdose does not cause diabetic ketoacidosis.

High blood glucose levels, not insulin overdose, cause diabetic neuropathy (nerve damage) and diabetic retinopathy (retina damage).

8.3 b) Apply direct pressure with a sterile dressing

The first step to treat a wound with significant bleeding is to apply pressure to the wound. This is done by placing a clean cloth or sterile gauze on the wound and applying firm pressure with the hand. The pressure helps to stop the bleeding by allowing the blood to clot. Maintain pressure on the wound for several minutes or until the bleeding stops.

8.4 b) Give the patient a sugary drink

The patient is wearing a diabetic medical bracelet, which means she has diabetes. The symptoms of fast heart rate and rapid breathing are consistent with insulin shock, which occurs when a diabetic takes too much insulin and their blood glucose levels fall too low.

If the patient can swallow, you should give them a drink containing sugar, such as orange juice, cola, or sugar dissolved in water. This will bring their blood glucose levels back up to normal. The patient will also require emergency medical attention.

If in doubt, give the patient sugar anyway. A patient with high blood sugar (hyperglycemia) can withstand the extra sugar whereas a patient with hypoglycemia needs sugar immediately to prevent possible brain damage or death.

8.5 c) unconscious but breathing normally

The recovery position is for people who are unconscious but still breathing. The position keeps their airway open and prevents choking.

The other options (breathing abnormally, cardiac arrest, and unconscious and not breathing) require CPR instead.

8.6 d) poisoning

Activated charcoal is used to treat cases of poisoning. It helps prevent the body from absorbing the poison.

8.7 a) Face, arm, speech and time

The acronym FAST helps to remember the symptoms of a stroke:

- F = Facial drooping
- A = Arm weakness
- S = Speech difficulties
- T = Time

8.8 b) 2

Chest compressions should be delivered at a rate of 100 to 120 per minute, or around two compressions per second.

8.9 d) percentage of body area affected by a burn

The rule of nines is a rapid method to estimate the percentage of the body's surface area affected by burns. It divides the body into sections, allowing for a quick estimation of the extent of burn injury.

In adults, the surface area is allocated as follows:

- Left arm: 9%
- Right arm: 9%
- Head and neck: 9%
- Chest: 9%
- Abdomen: 9%
- Upper back: 9%
- Lower back: 9%
- Left leg: 18%
- Right leg: 18%
- Genitals: 1%

8.10 c) Put something soft under their head

Putting something soft under the head of a person having a seizure can protect the head from bumps.

Mouth-to-mouth breaths are for someone who is not breathing.

You should never try to hold down someone having a seizure as this can cause an injury.

You shouldn't put anything into the mouth of someone having a seizure as this can injure their teeth or the jaw.

8.11 c) Immobilizing the arm

The first aid for a snake bite is immobilisation with a bandage and splint. Immobilisation helps contain the venom within the bitten area and prevent it from moving to the vital organs. First, the bandage is applied, to slow the spread of the venom through the lymphatic and circulatory systems. Then the splint is applied to keep the bitten limb still, further discouraging the spread of the venom.

Applying a tourniquet is not recommended because it cuts off blood flow and can lead to severe tissue damage.

Applying ice to the injury is not recommended because it can cause further tissue damage.

Trying to suck the venom out of snake bite wounds is ineffective.

8.12 d) When the person refuses care

Never administer care to a casualty who explicitly refuses care. Casualties have the right to refuse first aid treatment.

8.13 **a) Anaphylactic shock**

The combination of hives (skin reaction), difficulty breathing, and sneezing strongly suggests anaphylaxis, a severe and potentially life-threatening allergic response. In anaphylaxis, the body reacts to an allergen by releasing chemicals that cause:

- Airway swelling and bronchospasm (trouble breathing)
- Skin symptoms like hives and itching
- Widespread vasodilation (drop in blood pressure)
- Sometimes sneezing or wheezing

Anaphylaxis is a medical emergency that requires immediate treatment, often with epinephrine (adrenaline).

Option b, heart attack, causes chest pain and shortness of breath, not hives and sneezing.

Option c, insulin overdose, can lead to hypoglycemia, causing symptoms like confusion, sweating, and tremors.

Option d, stroke, typically involves symptoms like weakness or numbness on one side of the body, slurred speech, and confusion.

8.14 **b) 2**

In CPR, the recommended chest compression depth for adults is 2 to 2.4 inches.

8.15 **b) Call 911 → start CPR → defibrillation**

The "chain of survival" is the sequence of events that maximizes the chances of survival from cardiac arrest. The correct sequence is:

1. Call 911 to get emergency services on their way
2. Start CPR to maintain circulation and oxygenation
3. Use defibrillation to restore a normal heart rhythm

8.16 **a) The center of the chest**

For chest compressions in CPR, the hands should be placed in the center of the chest. This location ensures effective compression of the heart to restore blood flow.

8.17 **b) Airway, breathing, and circulation**

In first aid, ABC stands for Airway, Breathing, and Circulation.

- Airway: Ensure the airway is open
- Breathing: Check the patient is breathing
- Circulation: Assess the patient's circulation. If necessary, begin CPR (chest compressions and rescue breaths).

8.18 **c) Loosely wrap his fingers in bandages**

When transporting a patient with frostbite, loosely wrap the affected area in bandages, clothing, or blankets. You can also tell the patient to keep the affected area next to their body, where it is warm.

Hot water or a heating pad risks burning the affected area, since the patient may not be able to feel the heat correctly.

Vigorous rubbing can damage the affected area since frostbitten tissue is delicate.

8.19 **b) Keep the person's head still and do not try to move it**

If you suspect someone has a head, neck, or back injury, you must keep the person still until emergency medical care arrives. Any movement could result in paralysis or death.

8.20 **a) cardiac arrest**

The chain of survival is a series of actions that, when performed in order, increase the likelihood of survival from cardiac arrest.

8.21 **b) 30 compressions followed by 2 breaths**

When performing CPR, give 30 chest compressions followed by 2 rescue breaths.

8.22 **c) Place a tourniquet over the elbow joint**

When someone is bleeding, applying a tourniquet should be a last resort. This is because tourniquets can permanently damage nerves, muscles, and blood vessels, and even result in the loss of the extremity. Therefore, tourniquets should only be used as a last resort when all other methods of controlling the bleeding have failed.

Furthermore, tourniquets should never be applied to a joint. Placing a tourniquet over a joint can reduce its effectiveness in stopping bleeding. It can also cause nerve, bone, and tissue damage.

8.23 **a) choking**

The Heimlich maneuver is an emergency procedure for upper airway obstructions (choking). By exerting pressure on the bottom of the diaphragm, the lungs are forced to expel air, dislodging the obstruction.

8.24 **d) Terbutaline, epinephrine, aminophylline, and albuterol**

Terbutaline, epinephrine, aminophylline, and albuterol are used for breathing emergencies such as asthma, COPD, and anaphylaxis. Terbutaline, aminophylline, and albuterol are bronchodilators that relax smooth muscles in the airways. Epinephrine is both a bronchodilator and a vasopressor and is commonly used in anaphylactic emergencies.

8.25 **b) A man who had knee replacement surgery three days ago and now has swelling and pain in his leg**

The patient has signs of deep vein thrombosis, caused by the knee replacement surgery. Deep vein thrombosis is serious because the blood clot could break loose and get stuck in the lungs, which is known as a pulmonary embolism. Therefore this patient should be seen first.

A temperature of 99.9°F is only a low-grade fever and is therefore not a priority.

8.26 **a) Diazepam**

Diazepam (known commonly as name Valium) can be used in an emergency to stop a seizure. Other drugs that can stop seizures are lorazepam, midazolam, and clonazepam. These drugs all belong to a class of medications called benzodiazepines.

Epinephrine (adrenaline) is used for anaphylaxis, cardiac arrest, and asthma attacks.

Nitroprusside is a vasodilator. It is used to reduce blood pressure in patients with hypertensive crisis.

Terbutaline is a bronchodilator. It is used to treat asthma and other breathing conditions.

8.27 a) Blue

Blue is the hospital emergency code for an adult medical emergency, usually cardiac or respiratory arrest.

Generally, the other hospital emergency codes are:

- Red: fire
- White: pediatric medical emergency
- Pink: infant abduction
- Purple: child abduction
- Yellow: bomb threat
- Gray: combative person
- Silver: a person with a weapon
- Orange: hazardous material spill

Content Area 9

Managing Communication

There are 15 questions in this content area.

9.1 When talking to children, use:
   a) abbreviations
   b) jargon
   c) simple words
   d) technical language

9.2 When interacting with blind patients, you should:
   a) narrate your actions
   b) provide written materials
   c) use an interpreter
   d) use simple language

9.3 When communicating with someone from a different culture, it is important to:
   a) make assumptions about their beliefs and values
   b) speak louder and slower to ensure understanding
   c) be respectful of their cultural differences
   d) avoid using humor, as it may be misinterpreted

Answers on page 111

9.4 For which type of patient would an interpreter be useful?
   a) Blind
   b) Intellectually disabled
   c) Non-English speaking
   d) Pediatric

9.5 Which mail type ensures a letter will arrive the next day?
   a) Express
   b) Ground
   c) Priority
   d) Transit

9.6 What is the standard font size for business letters?
   a) 10 pt
   b) 12 pt
   c) 14 pt
   d) 16 pt

9.7 Which of these is a correct dateline for a business letter?
   a) 8/20/2024
   b) Aug. 20 2024
   c) Aug. 20, 2024
   d) August 20, 2024

Answers on page 111

9.8 Which format is this letter in?

> Springfield Medical Centre
> 123 Main Street
> Belleville, Illinois 62223
> January 1, 2024
>
> 456 Hill Street
> Belleville, Illinois 62223
>
> Dear Mrs Jones,
>
>   I am writing to confirm your upcoming appointment with Dr. Ann Smith at Springfield Medical Center. The appointment is on February 3, 2024 at 2:30 PM.
>
>   Please arrive 15 minutes early to complete any necessary paperwork.
>
>   Yours sincerely,
>   John Doe

- a) Full block
- b) Modified block
- c) Semi block
- d) Simplified

9.9 Mail marked _____ should be left unopened and given to the physician.
- a) important
- b) open immediately
- c) personal
- d) urgent

9.10 When does Medicare allow stamped signatures?
- a) During major disasters or imminent emergencies
- b) For low-priority claims of small amounts
- c) For physicians unable to sign due to a disability
- d) For physicians with a high volume of patients

Answers on page 111

9.11 What is the size of legal paper?
  a) 8.3×11.3 inches
  b) 8.3×14.3 inches
  c) 8.5×11 inches
  d) 8.5×14 inches

9.12 When answering the phone, you should state your name and:
  a) "How are you today?"
  b) the name of your facility
  c) your facility's opening hours
  d) your phone number

9.13 What term means sending medication orders and treatment instructions electronically instead of on paper charts?
  a) Computerized physician order entry
  b) Digital treatment instruction transfer
  c) Electronic medical record
  d) Electronic order scripting

9.14 Which law requires safeguards when sending health information by email?
  a) CAN-SPAM Act
  b) Health Insurance Portability and Accountability Act (HIPAA)
  c) Occupational Safety and Health Act (OSHA)
  d) Privacy Act

9.15 Medical assistants are allowed to:
  a) call in new prescriptions
  b) call in prescription refills
  c) change a patient's dosage
  d) prescribe medication

Answers on page 112

ANSWERS

9.1 c) simple words

When talking to children, use simple, clear language they can easily understand.

9.2 a) narrate your actions

Narrating your actions helps blind patients to know what is happening.

9.3 c) be respectful of their cultural differences

Being respectful of cultural differences is crucial in communication. This involves being mindful of different customs, beliefs, and practices, and avoiding assumptions or stereotypes that might offend or misunderstand the other person.

9.4 c) Non-English speaking

Interpreters are used when patients have little ability to speak or understand English.

9.5 a) Express

Express is typically the fastest domestic mail service offered by carriers like USPS. It guarantees delivery the next day in most areas.

Ground is the slowest option and wouldn't guarantee next-day delivery.

Priority mail usually takes 1-3 business days and therefore doesn't guarantee next-day delivery.

Transit isn't a term for a standard mail service.

9.6 b) 12 pt

The standard font for business letters is Times New Roman, size 12 pt.

9.7 d) August 20, 2024

In a business letter, the dateline should contain the month (fully spelled out), day, and year.

9.8 b) Modified block

The letter is in the modified-block format. In this style, the sender's address, date, and closing are centered or right-aligned, while the recipient's address and the body of the letter are left-aligned.

In the full-block, semi-block, and simplified letter styles, all lines are left-aligned.

9.9 c) personal

Medical assistants are often in charge of opening mail. However, mail marked "personal" or "confidential" should be left unopened and given directly to the recipient.

9.10 c) For physicians unable to sign due to a disability

Medicare requires signatures to be handwritten or electronic. The only exception is if someone has a physical disability that prevents them from signing their name. In this case, Medicare allows a stamped signature.

9.11 d) 8.5×14 inches

Legal paper measures 8.5 by 14 inches and letter paper measures 8.5 by 11 inches.

9.12 **b) the name of your facility**

When answering the phone, you should say your name and the name of your facility. This helps immediately inform the caller who they are speaking to and the organization they have reached.

9.13 **a) Computerized physician order entry**

Computerized provider order entry (CPOE) means entering and sending treatment instructions (including medication orders and laboratory requisitions) via computer rather than paper, fax, or telephone.

9.14 **b) Health Insurance Portability and Accountability Act (HIPAA)**

The Health Insurance Portability and Accountability Act (HIPAA) requires safeguards to protect health information, including health information sent by email.

9.15 **b) call in prescription refills**

In California, medical assistants can call in prescription refills under the physician's supervision. The medication refills must have no changes in the dosage levels.

Medical assistants cannot prescribe medication, call in new prescriptions, or change a patient's dosage. These are the responsibilities of the physician.

Index

ABC in first aid, 99
acetaminophen, 80
activated charcoal, 97
administering medications, 81–83
admission (ADM), 18
aerosol, 79
afebrile, 32
after visit summary, 92
aftercare instruction, 91
albuterol, 100
aminophylline, 100
Anadrol, 78
anaphylactic shock, 98
anesthetic, 79
antibiotic, 80, 92
antiemetic, 77
antihistamine, 79
anxiety, 22
apical pulse, 34
Aplisol, 46
appointment scheduling, 11
aspirin, 26
atrial flutter, 55
audiogram, 52
axillary temperature, 33

Bazett formula, 54
bilirubin, 45
bleeding, 96
blindness, 107
blood draw, 90
blood pressure, 32, 33

BMI, 36
body mass index, 32
body temperature, 35
bradycardia, 31
burn, 98

CAGE questionnaire, 23
California, 82
capillary puncture, 49
cardiac arrest, 100
cardiac treadmill stress test, 58
care instruction, 91
chain of survival, 99, 100
check, 11, 12
chief complaint, 24
children, 107
coinsurance, 17
colorectal cancer screening, 12
computerized provider order entry (CPOE), 110
convulsion, 101
copay, 16, 17
CPR, 97–100
crash cart, 100
credit card, 11, 12
cryosurgery, 91
culture, 107
Cushing syndrome, 48

date of birth, 17
dateline, 108
decibels, 52

deltoids, 81
diabetes, 97
diabetic shock, 96
diastolic blood pressure, 33
diazepam, 101
digoxin, 78
discharge instructions, 91, 92
discharge summary report, 93
diuretic, 79
dorsalis pedis pulse, 33
dressing pack, 22
dyspnea, 31

ear irrigation, 50, 51
ECG, 51, 53–61
ECG artifacts, 62
ECG electrodes, 54, 57, 59
ECG lead colors, 59, 60
ECG leads, 53–55, 57, 58, 60, 61
Einthoven triangle, 54
emergency, 11
emergency code, 101
Emergency Medical Treatment and Labor Act (EMTALA), 15
epinephrine, 100
extended-release tablet, 82

FAST, 97
fasting, 11
femoral pulse, 36
fever, 31
filing, 10
filing systems, 10
finger puncture, 49
first aid, 98–100
font size, 108
Fowler's position, 26
frostbite, 99

GAD-7, 22
generic drugs, 77
glucose, 50
glucose point-of-care testing, 49
glycemia, 49

haloperidol, 78

HbA1c, 48
health screening questionnaire, 24
hearing loss, 53
heart attack, 96
heart disease, 91
heart rate, 34
Heimlich maneuver, 100
HIPAA, 110
HIPAA Notice of Privacy Practices, 18
history and physical (H&P), 25
human chorionic gonadotropin, 46, 47
hyperkalemia, 79
hypertension, 30
hypoxemia, 30

ibuprofen, 26
immunity, 74
influenza, 75
inhalation, 79
injection, 82
insurance, 11, 16
interpreter, 108
intramuscular injection, 75, 76, 81, 83
Ishihara test, 51
Ishiwara test, 51

jaundice, 50, 91

LA electrode, 57
LDL, 78
lead I, 56
lead II, 61
lead III, 55
legal paper, 110
letter formats, 109
levothyroxine, 74
Lewis lead method, 55
lisinopril, 79
lithium, 78
lithotomy, 25

mail, 108, 109
mammogram, 12
median cubital vein, 43
medical history, 10

Medicare, 16, 109
Medicare Beneficiary Identifier, 17
medication, 23, 26
medication administration record (MAR) chart, 26
medication reconciliation, 23
midstream urine, 48
MMR, 77
MMR vaccine, 75
modified block, 109
myopia, 45, 52

nasopharyngeal swab, 47
nearsightedness, 52
neck injury, 99
needle disposal, 81
nitroglycerin, 78
Noots tank, 50
normal hearing range, 53
normal range, 32
not sufficient funds (NSF), 11
NPH insulin, 82

orthopnea, 31
otitis, 45
otoscope, 51
oxygen, 32

patient history, 10
patient identification, 22
peak flow meter, 48
peak flow rate, 48, 50
peak flow test, 49
peak flow zone system, 49
personal mail, 109
pharmacy abbreviation, 80
phlebotomy, 22, 42–45, 53
phlebotomy complications, 43, 44
phone etiquette, 110
photo identification, 18
photosensitive, 45
PHQ-9, 21
point-of-care testing, 49
popliteal pulse, 35
PPD test, 46

pregnancy strips, 47, 49
pronouns, 21
pulse oximeter, 33
pulse oximetry, 34, 35, 45
pulse pressure, 33
punch biopsy, 22

QT interval, 60

radial artery, 36
rapid strep test, 47
recovery position, 97
rectal temperature, 36
respiratory rate, 33
rhythm strip, 61
rotavirus, 76
rule of nines, 98

saturation of peripheral oxygen, 36
schizophrenia, 24
screening questions, 22–24
seizure, 98, 101
signature, 109
sitting position, 37
six rights of medication administration, 81
snake bite, 98
Snellen chart, 52
SOAP, 12, 23
sound frequency, 52
sphygmomanometer, 32
spironolactone, 79
staples, 90
statins, 78
stress, 21
stridor, 30
stroke, 97
subcutaneous injection, 80, 82
supine position, 25
suppository, 77
sutures, 90
systolic blood pressure, 34

tachycardia, 31, 56
tachypnea, 31
Tdap, 74, 75

temporal artery, 34
terbutaline, 100
tetanus, 11
thermometer, 37
throat swab, 46
tinnitus, 45
tourniquet, 43, 44
triage, 101
Tubersol, 46
tuning fork, 53
tympanic temperature, 34

units, 50
urinary tract infection, 91
urine collection, 47, 48

V1 electrode, 54
vaccination, 74–77
Vaccine Information Statement, 76
varicella, 75, 76
vasodilator, 77
vision, 52
vital slgns, 37

warfarin, 26
weight, 36
wheelchair, 35
wristband, 17, 18

Z-track method, 81

Top tips for study success

1   **Stay organised**
Keep your study area clean and organized. A clutter-free space can improve focus and productivity.

2   **Find your optimal study time**
Identify the time of day when you are most alert and focused, and schedule your most challenging tasks during that period.

3   **Set clear goals**
Define what you want to achieve in each study session. Having specific goals helps you stay focused and motivated.

4   **Create a schedule**
Establish a study schedule that aligns with your daily routine. Make your schedule clear to friends and family.

5   **Break it down**
Break your study material into smaller, manageable chunks. This makes it easier to understand and remember.

6   **Teach someone else**
Reinforce your knowledge by explaining what you've learned to someone else.

7   **Use different resources**
Explore various learning resources such as textbooks, websites, and videos to gain a well-rounded understanding of topics.

8   **Take regular breaks**
Take a break from studying every thirty minutes or so. Breaks help prevent burnout and improve concentration.

9   **Use memory techniques**
Experiment with mnemonic devices, flashcards, mind maps, or other memory aids to enhance retention.

10   **Reward yourself**
Once you've finished a study session, reward yourself. Try taking a long bath, listening to music, or watching a movie.